Can I talk you out of breastfeeding?

A quick read on everything that can be challenging about breastfeeding

Sophia Felder, FNP, IBCLC

Contents

Introduction:

There is a patriarchal culture in lactation medicine that I wish would die out; interactions with healthcare providers function under the assumption that if we warn you too much about how challenging it can be, you simply will choose not. The assumption is that parents will be overwhelmed with too much information, or back down from the fight. The unspoken rule is that we should keep this information from you and just tell you what to do as problems arise or keep you on a "need to know" basis. I loathe such a patronizing attitude and aim to be a part of the movement that changes that.

It has not been my experience that parents shrink away from a challenge. In fact, I see them work harder to get feeding to work than they have at anything else, in their entire life. Consequently, I am here to inform you of the ways in which lactation can be difficult and affect your life. So, the question is: can I talk you out of breastfeeding? I believe you will still try because knowledge is empowering. The more you know about it the more likely you are to succeed. The steep learning curve that happens when you have your first baby is currently too steep, especially for sleep deprived and vulnerable new parents. My aim is to flatten that learning curve and bring you more education about as many aspects of lactating as I can think of. Hopefully, I will catch you before or during pregnancy, so you are not trying to master such a hard topic while you are trying to recover from childbirth and adjust to your new role as a parent. The truth is that this is a journey full of many obstacles, even when things go well. However, we can do hard things!

Most other breastfeeding books I have found have been a generalized instruction manual that falls short of including the many variations that exist in lactation, and parenting. If they discuss issues it is downplayed, and the issues addressed are not all-encompassing of the real-life issues that modern parents face. This is not that type of book. You will not find rosy and peaceful expectations here. I will try to be inclusive of all people. I will not just reduce explanations to cute expressions, but actually explain the "why" behind struggles, and in some areas give suggestions, and options.

That being said, I do not want you to start reading this book with the expectation that I will give you solutions to all of these problems, because that would be unjust. If you face these problems you and your baby deserve personalized care, and thorough assessments from a professional. A book will never be able to give you all the answers because troubleshooting involves creativity and critical thinking. I am writing to open your eyes to the hard truths about lactating, and to remind you that help is available. This is in no way meant to scare you or discourage you from your feeding goals, and my title is tongue-in-cheek; I simply wish to explore the harsh realities so that you can enter the feeding relationship from an informed space. I believe by writing this book, I am engaging in my responsibility to deliver on the unmet needs of the population I serve.

I am here to tell you as a woman who has experienced many of the challenges with breastfeeding and pumping for my own children, and as a professional who works with parents every day who are struggling, that most classes and books are not providing a fair portrayal of all the nuances and struggles of feeding relationships. Nevertheless, many of us persisted; and you can too! At the same time, I want your persistence to be with better support and education behind it.

I have met too many parents in the last decade who have uttered "I never knew this," or "No one ever told me." Even beneath the joking request of "Can I take you home with me?" I hear the hidden message; parents are craving a different and more thorough education. What is available is leaving them wanting. I believe the tides are turning in healthcare, and the new expectation should be receiving education from your providers in order to engage in a shared-decision making process. We are leaving behind the days of patriarchal medicine, where the provider just tells you what to do, and does not educate you. This book is my contribution to that change.

I prefer to take what I believe is a more practical approach.

Let us acknowledge that this journey can be hard. I can educate, nurture, and encourage you despite that. I can help you face your fears and push through, because it can be a special experience even with the hurdles. Lactation is a complicated and nuanced experience and parents deserve so much more than a "how to" manual. Though, I do include some practical tips and a list of resources at the end of the book. Some tips are about many common struggles of parenting a newborn because this stage is hard, and you deserve as many helpful tips as you can get. I may even deviate a little bit here and there because it is hard for me to talk about parenting a newborn without including everything.

I am heavy on the science and medical knowledge, some would argue too much, because I want you to understand how your body and your baby's body will communicate through bodily functions and feelings, and the body will tell you the truth. You will hear the theme running through the text, "The body does not lie." People who like to be over-informed and know everything possible, will love it. So, I realize this will not be everyone's cup of tea. If information overwhelms you, you might want to read it in small chunks.

My main desire is for this book to make you aware of all of the challenges and possibilities of feeding, so that they do not come as a huge shock when you face them. Hopefully, this will make us all more empathetic to new parents in general, because we never know what they are facing. I include many things which people usually do not include when they teach about feeding, because I am always thorough. Also, some nuances may appear like redundancies. I did not delete my tangents or redundancies, because doing so would not be bringing you my authentic self. Ultimately, I want you to be a more informed and more confident parent. Hopefully, this book will be a great contributing factor to you becoming one.

About Me:

On a personal level, I have endured many challenges with breastfeeding and that has made me a more compassionate caregiver. I have had low supply, latch pain, thrush, tongue-tied babies, used nipple shields, pumped, taken medications, ingested herbs, used a supplemental nursing system, returned to work, suffered blisters, endured infections, and managed clogged ducts. I have fought this fight three times. I have been there, done that, and bought the gadget.

I believe now that my breastfeeding problems were a gift to me. I have a heart of service and want to use my gifts to help others. I was especially gifted sympathy for those struggling with breastfeeding. I deeply and personally know how it is such a vulnerable and special time. I have felt the strong and innate drive to fight through challenges to just feed my child. I have felt the heartache of failing.

Professionally, I am a Family Nurse Practitioner and an Internationally Board-Certified Lactation Consultant. I have a Bachelor of Science in Psychology, Bachelor of Science in Nursing, and Master of Science in Nursing. I have worked in Maternal-Infant Health since 2012, and breastfeeding support has always been part of my work; in 2018 I decided to make breastfeeding medicine a focus of my practice. After countless parents have expressed gratitude and appreciation for my candor and for educating them, I figured I have something to offer.

I work to be a part of the professional and modern parenting communities! I want to know what is working for parents right now! The breastfeeding industry is expanding so quickly research cannot keep up! I strive to provide evidence-based care, and sometimes all that I have is anecdotes. This is the current reality of the fast-paced world we live in. I do my best to balance that and use my best clinical judgement. Given all that information, I believe that I can help you. I want to help you. Simply, to help you through this time is my honor.

Disclaimer
This book is intended for educational and entertainment purposes only and does not replace medical advice following a thorough and detailed assessment by an appropriately credentialed provider. Reading this book does not establish a patient-provider relationship. The author disclaims any liability of outcomes based on the information provided in this book and expects all readers needing professional assistance to seek it in a timely and appropriate manner.

Trigger Warning:
This book contains upsetting and disturbing content that can be triggering. Topics include sexual abuse, domestic abuse, infant loss, labor trauma, and several others that can be upsetting. Know that this book goes into deep uncomfortable topics that are not often discussed in how they relate to the feeding experience. I found it important to include these topics because my book is heavily mental health focused. I have it peppered throughout the book, as well as a section focusing on it. If you have been through trauma, make sure you are in a safe space when reading, and with your support system easily accessible.

Can I talk you out of breastfeeding?

Sophia Felder, FNP, IBCLC

Chapters

The Female Parent

This is that part of the book that is a bit heavy in the medical jargon and information. If you do not care for medical technical information feel free to skip to the next chapter, or circle back to this later.

Breast development and other changes in the body

Your breast or mamma development begins in utero when you are in your mother's womb. Many things that influence the mammary tissue development, like your mother's diet and your genetic make-up, are outside of your control. From in-utero development to puberty, there are little to no changes to the breast tissue.

Right before puberty, or the first stage of puberty, there are breast buds developing. During puberty, your mammae develop further by filling out into a more rounded shape with fat and mammary tissue. This is to eventually be able to feed a baby, but this is not the final stage of mammary development. During puberty is another time when things are largely outside of our control. We typically follow the diet and lifestyle that our parents set up for us. During this developmental phase it is ideal to eat healthy, get exercise, and have a healthy body fat percentage. This helps regulate hormones in order to optimize breast tissue growth.

Additionally, many healthcare providers allow pubescent young females to skip periods on birth control. However, every month that you go through your hormonal cycles there is important mammary tissue development taking place. I believe knowing this, we can deduce that disrupting that breast growth monthly by suppressing the cycle with birth control in puberty can potentially be a risk factor for low supply when you start having babies.

Biologically the optimal time to create offspring and thus

feed them is when we are young, almost directly following the pubertal stage of breast development and the beginning of menstrual cycles, and when the hips are wide enough to pass a newborn through. Ideally, this is followed with many pregnancies. Younger females rarely ever have milk supply issues. By pointing out this biological norm, I am not encouraging teenagers to get pregnant, as there is obviously much more to consider in family planning than milk production.

While younger age makes you less likely to have supply issues, you will often see advanced maternal age a risk factor for low supply or having difficulty with building a milk supply. This is often when a female has a first-time pregnancy over the age of 35, and has an underlying hormonal health condition. The body will stop putting energy into mammary tissue development if you are not procreating during the optimal biological time frame. The tissues needed to make milk start to involute, and those tissues that remain are less sensitive to the hormonal receptors. Females who have had many babies and are older have the benefit of having grown mammary tissue with each pregnancy and are less at risk for supply issues. This is true even when the pregnancy does not reach viability. That being said, rarely is age alone a strong indicator for risk of low supply. Many times, the hormones of pregnancy are able to encourage enough growth of milk making glandular tissue needed to make a full supply.

Pregnancy is beneficial to supply because during pregnancy breasts grow and change, yet again. Some refer to pregnancy as the last stage of puberty for females. Hormonal and structural changes lead to long term permanent development that prepares your mammae to feed a baby. This is the second to last stage of development in as far as growing to feed offspring, because further development happens after the baby is born. This is not, however, the last time that the mammary structures will change. Your chest will never be the same. Despite the pervasive myth surrounding lactation and chest changes, you cannot blame it for the eventual sagging of breasts; that happens because of the changes during pregnancy! Whether you plan to feed your own milk or not, during pregnancy your body will prepare as if you are. With each pregnancy, even more glandular development occurs. That being said, pregnancy is not required to be able to nurse a child. The framework is there after puberty, pregnancy just makes the tissues multiply and increases their sensitivity to lactation hormones.

Adoptive and same-sex female partners are often able to bring in a partial milk supply for babies they did not carry in their own womb. Frequent suckling or pumping will encourage breast tissue changes because we are biologically programmed to help our offspring survive, even in the absence of the biological female parent. This is also why men are able to produce some milk. Our bodies want our offspring to have every chance at survival possible. The more caretakers that can make milk, the better. Pregnancy helps but does not guarantee a full supply, nor does not being pregnant mean you cannot make milk. The body is complicated like that. If you look at it from a lens of species survival and historical normalcy of villages raising children, rather than just one or two parents, this makes more sense.

The development of mammary tissue is also complicated by the influences of environmental toxins on our endocrine system, we call these endocrine disruptors. Our endocrine system controls all of our hormones, including the ones that encourage mammary tissue growth. With more environmental toxin exposure in recent history, more females are more likely to suffer from chronic low supply because of insufficient tissue development, which is regulated by the endocrine system. These toxins are also causing an increase in other chronic health conditions. So, with the rise of chronic underlying health conditions, we also see a rise of chronic low supply. The assaults on the body begin before we are even formed, as the cells we are made of before conception can be influenced by these toxins. These affronts and disruptions to development may also occur during puberty and pregnancy, influencing the mammary tissue development again. Generational environmental toxin exposure and changes to family structures have been part of the challenge of breast-milk feeding success in recent history. Those who suffer from chronic low supply should be seeking chronic underlying health issues that might be treatable.

During pregnancy, your mammae should ideally increase in size and your nipples and areolas should get larger and darker. The breast will appear to have many more prominently visible veins. This is because the vascular system is growing there, too. More blood needs to be brought to the breast because this is what your milk is made from. The larger size is due to more fat being stored in the breast, as well as due to the further developed mammary glands taking up more space as they grow. If you wear a bra, you will likely need to get a larger one. The darker areola is so the baby can find the nipple more easily because their eyesight is poor at birth. Several openings or holes in the nipple become apparent as the ducts become patent to allow for the milk to flow out of the breast. Sometimes the holes open on the areola, but most develop openings on the nipple tip. The average amount of duct openings on the nipple is 9 to 12 holes, but you might have less than that or more than that. I have seen rare cases where breasts do not develop duct patency or openings to allow for the flow, and their milk stays trapped in the breast, and breastfeeding is not possible. You might also develop Montgomery glands; these are dark little bumps all around the areola. They excrete an oil which has a smell that attracts the baby and allows the baby to recognize where to find milk. Additionally, some people notice larger and darker chest hairs, especially around the areola when they are pregnant or lactating. Hormonal imbalances during your pregnancy can influence mammary gland development and thus eventually milk supply sufficiency, which we cover next. If your mammae do not change in these ways, this can be a red flag for concern.

While pregnant, females who are prone to developing cysts might grow new cysts on the ovaries or in the mammae. Finding these growths can be alarming, and for good reason. The hormones of pregnancy and lactation can cause cancerous growths in females, especially those who are genetically prone to them. While lactating some develop galactoceles, or milk filled cysts. Imaging on the breast will help determine if the growths are simple cysts or cancerous tumors. Imaging during pregnancy and while lactating is complicated, but not impossible. Generally, you should at least be able to get an ultrasound and then if needed a biopsy. Always bring it to the attention of your healthcare provider if you believe you have a new growth, stay familiar with how your chest feels, and keep doing self-exams.

The Academy of Breastfeeding Medicine (ABM) publishes up to date protocols for imaging on the lactating people, which should be your reference if you find yourself needing imaging. You might have to be the one to tell your provider about these protocols, or push for the imaging, as not all are lactation medicine savvy. Some providers believe, erroneously, that you have to wean before imaging can be done.

You start making milk (well, colostrum) while pregnant, and you might leak! When your milk transitions from colostrum to mature milk a few days after the baby is born, you will likely experience engorgement. You can also develop mammary tissue anywhere along your "milk lines" which go from your armpits to your groin. Imagine the teats on other mammals such as cats and dogs to get a visual. Be prepared for possible swelling, extra nipples, leaking, or engorgement to possibly develop along the milk line.

Engorgement is a combination of the milk volume increasing, as well as water around the milk glands, this creates an uncomfortable tightness over the skin. This is often what others refer to when they say they felt their milk "come-in." Engorgement might be worse with each child but tends to resolve more quickly.

It is important to note that these changes can occur with every pregnancy, even when the infant does not survive or does not go home with you. Parents who lose their infants to death, adoption, or are delivering a surrogate baby will still make milk.

It can be very alarming and upsetting to realize that your body is trying to make milk for a baby that is no longer there. Engorgement or transition to mature milk is unlikely to happen after first trimester losses, but mammary tissue development still occurs. If you lose your baby in the second or third trimester, or during labor and delivery, your body will still respond by trying to bring milk in. Each person responds differently to this, but for many it can be a second wave of heartache and intense emotional upset as the hormones rage. For many parents, weaning and suppressing the milk is what feels best to them for grieving and moving forward. For some parents, choosing to continue to make milk and then donating that milk is very healing. Only you will know what is the right answer for you.

The edema in the chest that is part of the engorgement can be made worse when you are given a lot of fluids during labor and delivery. You will also notice a surge of edema in your hands and feet 1 to 3 days after delivery. The fluid needs displaced with lymph massage in the direction away from the breast, and will not always move or feel relieved when you try to remove milk. It seems contrary but drinking a lot of water helps stabilize the fluids in the body, and your body will release the extra fluids more readily if it knows you are well-hydrated. The fluid that your body stored during pregnancy is shifting out to your circulation so that it can be filtered out of the body via the blood flow to the kidneys and then to the bladder and then excreted through urination.

This process takes several weeks because if the dramatic fluid retention were shed too quickly it would cause severe electrolyte imbalances, and those can be life threatening. If your body is struggling with re-balancing the fluids, you might get diuretics for a few days, which can speed up the process. Often being on diuretics or hypertension medications can cause a temporary dip in supply, as it causes the body to shed fluid rapidly which is counter-productive to making more milk. Most will rebound from this and go on to make a full supply once it is safe for them to stop their medications.

Returning to the topic of the milk line, as your armpits are a part of that, you can expect that they change too. Rather, the smell coming from the armpit. The smell you give off needs to be stronger so that the baby can easily identify you compared to other caregivers, and be able to find you more easily when their eyesight has not yet finely developed. The smell needs to draw them close to the mammae, so the armpit is a logical place with it being next to the milk source. This change in smell is especially pungent in the first few months after the baby comes. You can see how this is biologically beneficial, especially as the newborn's eyesight acuity further develops in the first several months postpartum. Do not be surprised if you need a stronger deodorant, stronger soap, and more frequent showers.

After engorgement resolves you will encounter more changes in your chest. The breasts will seem to soften and not feel full like they did in the early postpartum days. The first few weeks is a common time for parents to worry about milk seeming to dry up or go away. When this change couples up with cluster feeding many people quit, thinking they are not making enough milk. The mammae feeling full is actually a sign that they are not being drained well. They should soften after this initial engorgement period, and feel softer still, after each feeding; feeling fuller only briefly right before the next feeding as they have refilled between feeds. After supply regulation the breasts continue to get flatter and have a less full feeling. This is because the mammae transition from being a storage warehouse, where milk is always ready to feed with some extra to spare, to a feed on demand factory where the milk is made and pulled out of the breast as the infant nurses and requests it. The mammae are never empty because the milk making is on a slow and continual process, so even if a baby nurses for a long time and the breast feels soft there is still milk coming, it is just at a slower rate than at the beginning of the feed. These changes are normal and expected, and you can check in with your lactation consultant about signs of true low supply if the change worries you.

Many people who do not experience engorgement erroneously assume that their milk never came in. It is possible if you have a baby that feeds very frequently and drains the mammae very well that you might avoid engorgement discomfort, and does not necessarily indicate a low supply. Many cases of low supply are only perceived low supply and not true low supply. Professional assessment is critical if you suspect insufficient milk supply or a dip in supply.

During these first few days of nursing you will also experience a new sensation in the breasts called a "let-down." We call it this because the cycle of hormones involves the brain sending hormones to the mammae, and then the breasts send the milk to the baby, all in a downward cascade. It is triggered by the suckling baby or pump, and this signals the brain to allow for the letdown to occur, so it is a feedback loop. The letdown involves the muscles around the milk ducts squeezing the milk out in faster and stronger gushes.

The letdown is a physical and hormonal occurrence. Many describe it as tingling, burning, or itching. It is often accompanied by a strong overwhelming tiredness, thirst, and hunger. In fact, following the urge to eat and drink while nursing can result in greater milk output, which is just one example of how well the biological process is designed.

The letdown is often pleasurable, but not always. The hormone oxytocin is largely responsible for this mechanism. Oxytocin is also responsible for contractions, orgasms, and bonding. When the newborn is nursing and the oxytocin surges it tells the body the baby is on the outside now, so it is time to shrink the uterus and make the milk. Not all people feel their letdown, so do not be discouraged if you cannot. Some also experience it in more unique ways, such as shoulder tension or a sudden negative emotional reaction. Typically, the early weeks will be when you feel the letdown the strongest. As your body adjusts the sensations might completely go away or at least be less intense. You are likely to stop feeling them when you nurse for a long time or are nursing your second or third child.

Phantom letdowns are the sensations of letdown without the occurrence of milk-flow. People have reported experiencing these in pregnancy and up to several years after weaning. They can be startling when you do not expect them, and they may or may not come with a bit of leaking.

Your mammae will change again while you wean, and for months to years after weaning. Your breasts do get rather flat once you wean, but this is temporary as the mammary tissue involutes or shrivels up. A reconstruction takes place over many months; after pregnancy and breastfeeding your breasts are much different than before. This is what is meant to happen and not something to be feared. This will happen whether you have milk for days, months, or years. Your mammae should have changed many times by this point in your life, and then they do again during and after menopause.

It is also possible for post-menopausal females to re-lactate to help feed their grand-children, and it is expected in some cultures. While they might not achieve a full supply, it helps in the caretaking of babies; and, to me, is further proof that we are not meant to raise newborns alone.

Risks of low or insufficient supply

Most parents worry about making enough milk. This is the most common concern expressed by new parents in my experience. It might decrease your worry to know breastfeeding is not an "all-or-nothing" game. *Any* breastmilk provides *all* the benefits! Regardless, you should know if you have risk factors of low supply. Knowing your risk factors can help you determine if you should work closely with an IBCLC during and after pregnancy to help optimize your supply, and your lactation experience.

Risk factors for low supply include infertility, chronic hormonal conditions, experiencing the first time lactating, first pregnancy after 35 years old, greater than 5 years since your last baby, obesity or high body fat percentage, underdeveloped breasts (insufficient or hypoplastic glandular tissue), subsequent pregnancy while still lactating, and previous chest surgeries.

Infertility is often undiagnosed or underdiagnosed. Many patients I meet who have struggled with pregnancy are unaware that what they experienced is considered "infertility." For the purposes of risks of low supply we will define this as taking longer than 1 year to get pregnant, having multiple miscarriages, needing progesterone to stay pregnant, or requiring any fertility aids or medical intervention to get pregnant or maintain pregnancy.

Having infertility is considered a high risk for low supply. Many people struggling with infertility are never warned of this. It is cruel to me to wait until breastfeeding is happening, and they are their most vulnerable, to prepare patients for this possibility. I found it extremely important to include in this book, especially given the fact that infertility rates are climbing. This can be considered a chronic hormonal condition. Setting aside logistical reasons, I really do not want to see another person who has been repeatedly heartbroken by infertility taken by surprise and heartbroken yet again because their body is not doing what they expect it to do when they attempt breastfeeding. In an already unjust and crushing experience, the last thing people need is for this information to be withheld from them. In addition, infertility can make it hard for a person to trust their body and makes one more likely to accidentally self-sabotage breastfeeding when they are having high self-doubt without adequate support.

Other chronic hormonal conditions could include polycystic ovarian syndrome (PCOS), hirsutism, thyroid dysfunction, pituitary tumors, diabetes, gestational diabetes, endometriosis, obesity, and many others. Obesity is part of this puzzle, as fat cells hold onto hormones that can influence the entire hormonal system, and of course there is the question of whether or not an underlying chronic hormonal condition is causing the obesity. Additionally, females who are obese typically have a longer delay in milk coming in which leaves room for unintentional supply sabotaging in the early days postpartum. Underdeveloped breast tissue is often a symptom of having an underlying chronic hormonal health issue, and that may be masked by high body fat percentage because it makes the breasts appear large. A breast can be large because it is full of fat, and not because it is full of milk making glands.

Other than the hormonal concerns of a high body fat percentage, there are logistical concerns as well. It can be physically more difficult to get into comfortable nursing positions, and many products designed to help make nursing easier do not have larger people in mind. It can be harder to succeed because of the stigma associated with being overweight. Your providers might assume you are going to fail due to hormone dysregulation, or they might assume you are lazy or unmotivated. While this may not be personally true, it does play on your emotions when your healthcare team does not believe in your success. Having a supportive team and tools to make things logistically easier are critical to long term breastfeeding success.

Most of the hormonal low supply factors are explained due to breast development and breastfeeding being hormonally regulated. If your endocrine system is dysfunctional it is more likely to also malfunction when you ask it to regulate breastfeeding. Your hormones might even be "within normal range" yet not optimal. However, risk factors do not equal a definite problem! They just call for close monitoring and might require some extra work be done to build and maintain supply.

For some, milk never comes in or increases beyond a few milliliters. I have seen this happen despite having no apparent risk factors. If you are not producing ounces versus milliliters by the time baby is 2 to 3 weeks old, your milk is very unlikely to increase much beyond that; rare and extenuating circumstances not included. While you can maintain a breastfeeding relationship, it is harder to do and takes some creativity.

Many risk factors might just make your milk late to come in versus chronically low in supply. It may come in days 5 to 7 rather than the typical days 3 to 5. It is unusual and does not occur often, but some have reported milk not coming in until day 10-14. Extremely rare might be about 20 days postpartum, if you had a special circumstance like a rare type of cyst that delays hormonal changes needed to bring milk in. For most, after 2-3 weeks postpartum they are no longer hormonally primed to bring in milk, as crucial hormones diminish. It is important to allow a few weeks of attempting to breastfeed and pump to start to get a clear picture of the long-term supply possibilities. Most people have 4-6 weeks to build a supply once the milk comes in. After about 4-6 weeks the baby's volume needs stabilize, and some key hormones are reduced.

As mentioned above, breast milk production is also influenced by certain hormonal conditions. Complete suppression of supply can happen for multiple reasons related to hormonal regulation, as well. Breastfeeding through a pregnancy is an example of this and is its own discussion due to the hormonal changes that happen while pregnant. A brief exploration of some of the female hormonal regulation through the childbearing years will help paint the picture of how the hormones influence milk production.

Lactation suppresses ovulation for most, and this can serve to help naturally space out children. Of course, some people get pregnant easily while lactating so this cannot be considered a reliable form of birth control. Recommendations to space out children a minimum of 18 months helps you maintain a milk supply, lets your body heal, and gives you time to replenish nourishment storage between pregnancies. Having babies too close together automatically makes your pregnancy high risk because it increases your chances of several negative outcomes and complications. We have a lot of evidence that this is unsafe for both the female and the baby. Additionally, due to changes in the breasts during pregnancy it can take away the opportunity for an optimal breastfeeding experience with the older child. Close spacing risks are exacerbated when babies are delivered via cesarean, because this takes longer to completely heal from; it results in a temporarily weakened state of the uterus due to the incisional injury, and a higher risk of the placenta adhering dangerously deep into the uterine scar tissue. I will not go more in depth on that topic here, as it is outside the scope of this book.

The reasons that closely spaced pregnancies can result in an interference with breastfeeding an older child are due to supply decrease, and nipple sensitivity. While pregnant, estrogen and progesterone from the placenta suppresses mature milk. As the placenta forms in the early weeks you will make less and less milk. As the first trimester passes it will become colostrum again, due to the new placenta taking over your body's hormonal regulation so strongly. Unless you are lucky, this decrease in volume will mean you do not have enough milk to sustain your baby before 1 year of age. It might be possible if your first trimester overlaps with their 1-year birthday, or the nursling is over 1 year old and not requiring a large volume of milk. The placenta usually does not take over hormone regulation until around 12 weeks gestation. The older child can supplement his nutritional intake with alternative milks and high fat foods. The unborn baby is in no risk of being deprived of nutrients.

You do have the option to "dry nurse" through a pregnancy and then tandem feed your babies at the same time when the younger child is born. Dry nursing is continuing the nursing relationship despite minimal milk transfer. It will be up to your baby if they are willing to keep nursing with the decrease in flow and change in flavor, and up to you if you can tolerate the discomfort. The discomfort of "dry nursing" is due to the increased estrogen in pregnancy making your nipples overly sensitive and thus nursing potentially painful or irritating. Many people experience intense nursing aversion during pregnancy with these changes. You will still need to supplement with donor milk or formula if your baby is under 1 year old, as the lowered amounts will likely not be enough for optimal hydration and growth. It can be a challenge to keep a baby nursing when not much milk is there, and your baby might decide to wean regardless of your plans. They might return to the breast once the milk is flowing again, and this can help them feel connected to you when the baby is taking up so much of your attention.

There is also the possibility of being forced to wean abruptly if you have a high risk pregnancy that requires "pelvic rest" due to threat of premature delivery or a placenta that is attached in an unhealthy way. Pelvic rest will mean no nursing, no orgasms, and nothing be inserted into the vagina, and I will explain why. Pelvic rest is put in place to avoid contractions from oxytocin surges during orgasms, it also prevents the cervix from being irritated or having pressure put on it by things pushed into the vaginal canal. Oxytocin also surges when you have a letdown while your baby is nursing, so contractions can be triggered when you are nursing. There are certain conditions where this would be very unsafe. In general, most pregnancies can handle the oxytocin surges. If you are on pelvic rest, it is wise advice to wean. If you are not on pelvic rest and your provider suggests that you wean you might ask them to explain why or get a second opinion.

The placenta is the main driver of the supply changes during pregnancy, so, similarly to avoiding too closely spaced of pregnancies you also do not want to ingest any placenta after delivery due to its high progesterone content—it can suppress your milk! The delivery of the placenta causes a huge drop in progesterone, which is needed in order to have the huge spike in prolactin, which leads to the milk coming in. It is best to avoid re-introducing that progesterone into the body. No smoothies, no pills, no raw placenta steak, nothing! Your supply might be safe if you ingest it only immediately after delivery and not on an ongoing basis, or after 4-6 weeks postpartum once you have established that you have a good supply. Watch closely for supply changes when you ingest it, and if you continue to ingest it regularly. This is not the place to explore safety of placenta ingestion, I only want to touch on its effects on milk supply.

Comparably, if fragments of your placenta are retained in your uterus after delivery or you develop a uterine infection, this can cause a decreased supply or a delay in the milk coming in. Sometimes milk is much later to come in than is typical when the retained placenta is passed or removed within the first 2 to 3 weeks postpartum, but can then rebound to a full supply. Sometimes the retained placenta is noticed immediately after delivery, and a procedure has to be performed to get it out of the uterus. Retained or morbidly adherent placenta in one pregnancy makes you very high risk to experience it again in future pregnancies. The best thing you can do is monitor yourself for abnormal bleeding.

In order to know what irregular postpartum bleeding is, you must first know what is normal. For up to 8 weeks after the delivery of your baby you will bleed on and off to shed the uterine lining and clean out the womb. There will be a mix of blood, clots, discharge, and white blood cells. It is called lochia, and is many colors and textures. It typically starts as bright to dark red the first few days, then becomes pinkish brown for a few days to a few weeks, then white to yellow discharge will dominate. All the while it could be a mix of all three or go back and forth between types. The smell is usually odd to foul, but if it is consistently strongly foul you need to notify your provider. Small clots are okay, as long as there are not a large number of them, like more than 5-10 per 24 hours. Sometimes there are larger clots in the first 24 hours, but after that they should not be larger than a golf-ball. Often, clots form in the vaginal canal behind a full bladder which blocks the flow out of the vagina, and then they fall out once the vaginal canal is no longer being blocked as the bladder drains and lifts off of it. This means you will likely see some clots or surges in blood flow when you empty your bladder. You will want to call your doctor or midwife if you are bleeding bright red, have a strong foul odor, a fever, many small clots, clots larger than a golf-ball, or you are filling a large pad hourly (or more often). The bleeding will ebb and flow and tends to pick up if you are exerting yourself too much physically. It is almost like the body has a built-in way to say, "hey, you are doing too much!" You might not bleed as much or as long after a cesarean versus a vaginal birth, because they remove more of the uterine content in surgery than would naturally come out immediately after a vaginal delivery. You might not bleed for the entire 8 weeks, but you should be prepared that it might be off and on in that time frame.

If you need to start birth control the hormonal options can influence milk supply as well. Low dose progesterone-only options are typically safe for most, but non-hormonal options are the safest. Having limited options of birth control while nursing can be a challenge. A trial of the progesterone only mini-pill for a month can help determine how sensitive you are to the synthetic progesterone found in birth control. Avoid all types of birth control except barrier methods for the first 6 weeks postpartum in order to avoid interfering with milk supply. If a hormonal option like a shot, implant, or intrauterine device (IUD) is offered in the first 6 weeks and you want to establish breastfeeding then it is best practice to wait, and be sure to do a trial of a mini-pill first. Many hospitals still practice offering these options immediately postpartum, and this can ruin your supply before you even have a chance to build one up. After six weeks when the supply is more established you can do a trial of the mini-pill, and if it does not affect your supply you should be safe to stay on it or then get the longer lasting options like the shot, implant, or IUD. Those that are safe can still be detrimental to supply if started too early. The milk needs an opportunity to fully come in and be established before interfering with the hormonal cycles in the body. You should definitely avoid choosing birth control with estrogen, because that can dry you up completely, no matter how many months or years postpartum you are. The same is true of estrogen creams, which can be prescribed for conditions of the labia and vulva. Even a tubal ligation might result in tubal ligation syndrome—a symptom of which is low supply. Non-hormonal options like the copper intrauterine device and barrier methods pose the least risk to supply regulation. Those would be your best option until supply is established, and perhaps the entire time you are nursing if you find that your supply is sensitive to the hormonal options. All of this is actually not common knowledge amongst family and maternal health providers, and many will offer you birth control and suggest that the contraceptive method should not affect your supply, when in fact it does. While a birth control option might be safe, that does not mean it will not influence the hormones that regulate your milk production. There is a discrepancy between what the manufacturers claim and promote to providers versus the real lived experience of lactating people. Many IBCLCs are able to identify this trend, and it needs to be part of your thought process when choosing which birth control to use, and when.

Previous chest surgeries are another important risk factor worth discussing in depth, and not surprisingly are also partially hormonally mediated. Breastfeeding after chest surgery is most commonly discussed in reference to breastfeeding with breast implants. First to address is safety; and it is considered safe to breastfeed with breast implants. The likelihood for success after surgery is more intricately linked to the injury caused by incisions during surgery rather than the placement of the implant, which is what most people assume. If incisions during surgeries on the chest sever important nerves that help send signals from the breast to the brain you might find that when you need them to function for breast feeding you get diminished or absent signaling. If the brain does not get the physical signal that you have a frequently suckling baby, then it will not send the right hormonal cocktail to the breasts to then respond to the demand for milk. Numbness of the nipples can indicate that there will be diminished or absent signaling to the brain. Incisions can also cause scar tissue that blocks duct flow within the breast. This is true with any incision to the chest such as chest tubes, heart surgery, lung surgeries, biopsies, cyst removal, breast reductions and implants. The implant and incisions may also diminish your ability to sense breast fullness or your let-down sensation. The presence of the implants can also make breast compression and massage less effective or awkward, as the implant will be in the way. With breast augmentation the placement of the implant is less important than incision locations and what the breasts looked like before surgery, but if the implant is beneath the muscle it is less likely to impact breast-feeding.

It is possible in some cases for injuries to important nerves and tissues in the breast to heal by reconnecting or creating new connections. If it has been more than a few years since surgery this increases the chances that healing has occurred. It is generally understood that the longer the body has had to heal, the less likely the surgical history is to play a role in breastfeeding success. In some instances, people initially heal from surgeries in a way that does not impact lactation at all, regardless of the risk associated.

The breasts' development and appearance prior to surgery are important because they might be a clue to insufficient glandular tissue. When the breasts are dramatically asymmetrical, tubular, underdeveloped, or widely spaced these can be signs that the glandular breast tissue did not fully mature or proliferate. Your history of breast development and history of chest surgery are an important part of assessing your risk of having a low supply. When there is high risk for a low supply, such as in cases as this, we might suggest doing more than usual to help maximize supply in the early weeks postpartum.

Breast reduction surgery is the most common scenario where patients are falsely promised by the surgeon that there will be no future problem with lactation. My assumption is that they must not be following up on this claim, because this is far from the truth. Every lactation consultant cringes internally when they hear a patient has been told by the surgeon that lactation should not be an issue after reduction. It simply is not true, regardless of their skill. They damage and remove important tissues and nerves, especially when they cut around the areola. When it comes time to breastfeed the brain cannot get the signal it needs to know there is a baby that needs fed, because it cannot get the input from the suckling. They may even remove some of the milk making glands and the ducts where the milk flows. The scar tissue can also block the milk duct flow between the mammary glands and the nipple. If you are contemplating breast reduction and feel strongly about breastfeeding it is best to wait until you are done having children. Any surgery to the chest poses a risk to your supply, but none mentioned above have as high of a risk as breast reduction procedures.

Clearly, females who have mastectomies or large lumpectomies are at the greatest risk of supply concerns. It is possible if enough milk glands are left intact to still nurse on a breast that has had a partial mastectomy. If one breast is not surgically altered, it might be possible to nurse on that side. If the mastectomy is performed due to breast cancer, the cancer might return with the surge of hormones in pregnancy and lactation, causing the need for premature weaning. This might be a reason that your oncologists may suggest not attempting to breastfeed.

Having a history of breast cancer or mastectomy does not automatically mean that you cannot attempt to breastfeed, unless you have had a complete mastectomy of both breasts or your oncologist advises against it. This can be hard to face when you deliver in a breastfeeding friendly hospital, because breastfeeding will be repeatedly addressed due to scripts and protocols in place. After a reconstruction, you might be cleared to nurse using an SNS system (more on that system later). Deciding what to do is a decision best made with your healthcare team involved.

Sometimes people breastfeed their first child, but cancer prevents them from breastfeeding their other children. This might be due to needing surgery, needing chemotherapy, or being too high risk for cancer return. You will need to work with your oncology team to decide what is safest for you and your baby.

Under the same topic of scar tissue in the chest, we consider nipple piercings. This can have varied results. For some people, getting a nipple piercing causes scarring such that the duct flow is blocked, and they are unable to nurse or they have a slow flow. On the opposite end of this spectrum sometimes the extra holes that are created through the piercing are open to the milk flow and subsequently cause such a strong flow that it is a struggle for the baby to manage it. Some results fall somewhere in between, and some notice no interference to the relationship at all. Unfortunately, you just will not know until you try! It is critical, however, that piercings be removed from the nipple before nursing, to avoid a choking hazard.

Some other milk supply risk factors can also develop during labor and delivery, and immediately postpartum. It should come as no surprise at this point that the reasons are largely hormonal. These factors include induction, cesarean, premature delivery, maternal-infant separation, hypertension, an intravenous magnesium drip, epidural pain control, certain medications, retained placental fragments, too much blood loss, not removing the milk frequently enough in the first few days, mood instability, and birth injuries in the infant.

Please do not refuse medical intervention for the sake of your milk supply as they are often needed to keep you and your baby alive and free from more serious injury; just be aware that some interventions can influence breastfeeding and you will need to be extra diligent and work closely with an IBCLC. Most of these risk factors just require a greater effort in the early days, and may cause a delay in milk, but are not the cause of chronic supply issues.

Again, we largely look to hormonal regulation. When things get complicated during labor and delivery, we must intervene with procedures and drugs. These are needed, a modern medical miracle, and should be appreciated. However, they do interfere with our hormones a bit, and can leave the body confused for a few days. The shock of cesarean on the body often leads milk to come in a few days later for people who have the surgery, versus those who deliver vaginally. Birth injury in the baby is a separate topic that might occur during labor and delivery; however, we will cover it more in depth in the baby chapter. This section will continue to focus mostly on the female parent's body.

During labor you will likely be offered medications for pain management, and it is seldom fully disclosed that they risk interruption to the breastfeeding relationship. The pain options have opioids in them, and can cross the placenta. There are some studies showing babies are more sleepy after a laboring person gets pain medications during labor, which makes them less likely to nurse efficiently the first few hours after birth, when it is most critical that they do. Additionally, these medications increase the risk of needing a vacuum or forceps assisted delivery which might cause injury to the baby which influences how well they nurse. If the perineum needs stitching due to this the team might delay skin to skin to focus on you and your baby's injuries first. Often with pain medications the second stage of labor is longer than usual, which means more pushing. This can tire you and the baby out, making efficient nursing less likely in the first few hours postpartum. Epidurals usually come with a big bag of fluid prior, to avoid a dip in blood pressure that sometimes happens when you get one. More fluid can inflate baby's birth weight and cause worse edema for you postpartum, and worse edema usually comes with more swollen breasts, and that makes it harder for the milk to come out. Common reactions to epidurals are nausea, itching, vomiting, and an increase in temperature.

There is often confusion and myth surrounding epidurals, as well as differing professional opinions. Most people are also unaware that there are spinal versus epidural techniques, and use these terms interchangeably when they are different forms of anesthesia. The American College of Obstetrics and Gynecology (ACOG) says that the medications of epidurals can cross into the placenta, and are sometimes found in breastmilk. If you are a candidate for epidural, a needle will go into your spinal fluid between the bones, and the needle is removed and in it's place a small tube is left, called a catheter. The small tube delivers medication into the epidural space; the medication can have various effects but the main one is blocking pain signals. The epidural is placed in a space that is around the spinal cord. The space is where some spinal fluid is held, if spinal fluid is leaking out of this space it is not normal. Spinal anesthesia goes deeper into the spinal fluid space, giving a deeper intensity and is a single injection versus a continuous tube placement. Sometimes spinals and epidurals are both done at the same time. The types of epidurals and spinals available will depend on your delivery method and hospital, but some completely numb and deaden your legs while others make it possible to be pain free but still able to walk or move in the bed.

Epidurals also lead to the risk of needing a blood patch. While this sounds scary and like it involves blood, it does not. It is just oddly named. Your anesthesia team would go patch the small hole left by the epidural needle, to stop the spinal fluid from leaking. The reason you might want this done is because of something called a spinal headache. If you have a severe headache following an epidural, it might be because the hole created by the needle has not closed properly. The leaking of the spinal fluid alters the pressure in the brain and spine and you get a headache because your body is trying to tell you there is a problem. This can influence breastfeeding because the headache is often severe, and laying down seems to help. This can make breastfeeding feel awkward, or you might be in so much pain you do not care about breastfeeding. Getting it fixed quickly will be in your best interest if it does not resolve on its own within a few days. Other more rare risks of spinals or epidurals include bruising, infection, or abscess.

Many laboring people, obviously, get epidurals and go on to have no issues with breastfeeding. The information provided here is not intended to scare you away from them, it is just to make sure that you are getting as much information as you need in order to make a fully informed decision.

Other pain management options might include nitrous oxide gas. This is compatible with breastfeeding, as it leaves the body within minutes and insignificant amounts remain in the blood after the therapy is stopped. There is no evidence that it passes into milk.

Other issues in the labor and delivery period can arise, even with an unmedicated delivery. For a few hours after delivery many people experience violent shaking of their whole body off and on, and few are warned that this might happen. This can make you afraid to hold your baby, but it should still be safe to be skin to skin with a support person close by. We are unsure what causes this shaking, but it is likely the shock of the pain, the huge hormonal shifts, and the blood loss. If you do not know it might be coming it can be a very scary experience and feels scary even when you are warned beforehand because the body feels out of control. Some people mistakenly attribute this to epidural, but this happens even in people who do not get one.

Even when things go well during labor and delivery, most people experience huge mood shifts the first few weeks postpartum due to the dramatic lifestyle changes, hormonal changes, and sleep deprivation. It is normal to be weepy, a bit anxious for baby's safety, delirious, and exhausted. It is normal to go through a stage of grief, even when you were looking forward to this new change, you still grieve the past.

Your grief might be for your old self, your old life, how your romantic relationship used to be, how your body used to look, how much independence you had, your plans for delivery, your plans for feeding, what you thought your baby would be like, and many other aspects of parenthood making your life different, or different than you planned. When people fight that or are unaware that it is normal it can cause them to be hard on themselves, wonder if they are a bad parent, or cause them to make poor decisions around what is best for themselves, and best for the breastfeeding relationship. Grieving these things does not make you a bad parent, it makes you a normal human.

When a baby has an injury, is premature, or has a chronic health condition it introduces another set of challenges that we touch more on later. Prematurity is important in the female's risk factors due to them missing the last weeks or months of mammary tissue development, missing early breastfeeding relationship interactions, as well as the emotional trauma of the experience. Typically, the events surrounding premature delivery and a NICU stay are incredibly stressful and unexpected. It feels very unnatural and upsetting to the parent to be separated from their infant.

Regardless of gestation at delivery, when you have a particularly challenging birth it is tempting to try to rest as much as possible and let family take over feedings. It is also possible that maternal conditions might require separation, or keep someone too sleepy or ill to frequently stimulate their breasts. Baby also needs a lot of rest, because being born is hard work. They might be very sleepy at the breast, and you will have to work to keep them awake to eat enough.

You can keep baby awake by tickling them, changing positions, taking burp breaks, rubbing them with a cool wet cloth, changing their diaper, or compressing the breast to increase flow. They might even need supplementing if they cannot stay awake long enough to get an adequate feed.

Not removing the milk often enough or efficiently enough in the early postpartum days can be detrimental to supply. This is one of the risk factors that can cause chronic low supply. It is best to drain the breast as much as possible every 2-3 hours and to have no more than a single occurrence of a longer stretch than that every 24 hours; generally we can get away with one stretch of 4 to 6 hours for rest. The baby will still need to eat while we rest, until they are old enough and gaining weight well enough. Outside of that, expect 8 to 12 times in 24 hours of milk removal, by pumping or nursing. This can be every 5 to 60 minutes when baby is cluster feeding, or every 2 to 3 hours for the longer stretches between feeds. Gradually as the milk supply is established your baby will stop cluster feeding so often and go for longer stretches between feeds more consistently. If the baby is not draining the breast, you will need to hand express or pump to do so. When milk supply is more established, you can pump or nurse less often.

If you are mostly pumping, it can be tempting to pump less often when you notice that you get more pumped milk out if you wait more hours, but this can backfire. When you are at capacity, or the most full, you get the most milk that you can make in one sitting. For most people this happens in 4-6 hours. When you allow the breast to fill without frequent draining, you are signaling to your body that you want less milk. With the sensation of fullness there is a hormone produced that signals the body to reduce over-all supply. So, while you would initially see more milk per pump, your daily pump amounts would gradually decline. Frequency is more important to increasing supply, even when the initial amounts pumped are low. The frequent milk removal signals to the body that you want more milk. Due to the hormonal signaling, frequency and small pump sessions are superior to boosting supply than longer stretches between sessions with initially larger volumes. It is better to pump 8 times per day for 5 minutes than it would be to pump once per day for 40 minutes. This frequency more closely mimics baby's natural feeding, as newborns tend to eat frequently and in an erratic pattern, or cluster-feed.

The reduction of baby's cluster feeding patterns coincides with our milk regulation hormonal patterns, first around 6 weeks and then again around 12 weeks. The erratic nursing pattern, or lack of a real pattern, is how the baby works with your body in tandem to continue to boost the supply the first 6 weeks. The cluster feeding and the sporadic nursing keep the breasts at a low volume compared to capacity, and this is what signals to the body to keep increasing the supply. This is why most lactation professionals discourage parents from putting a breastfed baby on a schedule. This is logistically challenging, as it makes planning around nursing tricky when there is lack of a schedule. As their schedule regulates or becomes more predictable so does the milk because your body starts to get the signal that the baby is more content. If they never seem satisfied the first 4 to 6 weeks, it is because it is their job to act that way. This is part of the design of boosting the supply. Even bottle-fed babies will try to follow these instincts and cluster feed frequently the first 4-6 weeks. Their behavior, as such, is not the best or only indicator of adequate milk supply or transfer. The best indicators are diaper output and weight gain.

Even if it seems they are never satisfied, it is important to note that at times they actually are. To know if a baby is sometimes content, you will see their body give you clues. If they are truly never content, this might be a red flag and cause for concern. A content baby usually has open and relaxed hands, gets sleepy and drowsy at the breast after 10-15 minutes or more of nursing, their sucking starts to slow down, and they have good diaper output and weight gain. If they are nursing 30-45 minutes and coming off crying and upset, they may not be getting enough.

A common problem I see in the first few weeks postpartum with efficient milk removal is a simple issue of not offering both breasts every feeding. Many in-patient perinatal healthcare staff will erroneously advise, or parents assume, one breast per feeding is adequate. When milk volume is still low, a baby will generally get more volume if they take both breasts, and the supply will be more adequately stimulated.

As both breasts start to fill with mature milk, when you offer the first breast and it is its most full, then the initial 2-3 let-downs every 2-3 minutes are a fast flow and the baby gets most of the volume in the first 5-6 minutes. They will keep nursing past that to get more milk and to seek comfort. While on the first breast the baby dozes off as the rate of flow slows down. This does not mean they are done, or full. The baby will have gotten to the fatty hindmilk and drained the breast well if they are starting to doze off. This is when you should at least offer the second side. When you offer the second full breast, they get the faster flowing milk again, and are happy to drink more. This is how a baby gets more volume spending 10-15 minutes on each breast, rather than 20-30 minutes on one breast. This is not only beneficial to supply regulation but also reduces engorgement discomfort as well as baby's risks of jaundice, weight loss, inadequate gain, and poor blood sugar stabilization.

When a lactating person has a more abundant supply the baby might stop taking both sides at some of the feeds, or at all of them. It is helpful to always offer both, but do not expect them to always take both. There is usually no reason to worry if they do not always take both sides, but in the early days postpartum you should be consistently offering both sides so that the option is available.

Once supply is more established and capacity determined, you might find that your baby needs only one breast because each of your breasts can hold a full 5 ounce feed. You would in that case want them to finish the feed on one side to ensure they got to the fatty hind milk. This can be confusing or hard to guess if your baby needs one or both sides, so do not be afraid to go check in with a consultant to clarify what would be best for you and your baby.

There is no good blanket advice that will work for everyone, such as "10-15 minutes on each breast," because there is so much variation in capacity of breasts and efficiency of infants. Worrying about foremilk hindmilk balance and how it relates to offering both breasts usually only comes up if babies are struggling to gain weight, or if a parent has an over-supply; so it is not something that most parents will have to worry about.

There are so many other reasons why the demands of breastmilk supply establishment might not be met in the early days. If something happens where a parent is separated from their infant, or they are too ill to nurse or pump, then a plan needs to be made about how to protect their supply. Parents may be re-admitted to the hospital with a complication like pre-eclampsia or a uterine hemorrhage. Some hospitals separate a parent from their infant or need to put a parent in a medically induced coma. A lactating person might temporarily lose consciousness or lose physical custody. They may have a hard time choosing to nurse over bottle feeding when they have a spinal headache from their epidural and it makes positioning challenging. The list of possible complications is just too long to cover it all here.

You can (and should) make a plan with your partner, close family, or friends on how you would like your breastmilk supply protected if you are unable to do so yourself. Partners or other family members can work with the nursing and lactation team to express your milk on a schedule, even if you are physically unable to do it yourself. If baby is not with you, or you are unable to latch them, you still need to pump regularly. It is okay to ask the nurse to help with this.

An additional complication to consider on this topic is the risk factor of having too much blood loss, or hemorrhage, and how this can lead to chronic low supply. This causes a shock to the pituitary gland (one of the main glands in the brain that controls breast milk regulation), and some people do not overcome this shock. It is called "Sheehan's Syndrome." It can be helpful to review with your lactation consultant what your reported blood loss was, and especially if you needed a blood transfusion.

Risks for low supply might be mitigated by taking extra

effort to maximize supply in the last month of pregnancy and in the early weeks postpartum. Examples of this might be extra hand expressing, pumping, herbs, hormonal testing, or medications. Studies show that antenatal hand expression can boost postpartum supply. Having some expressed milk ready to feed can also help keep your baby's energy levels up and make them more efficient at the breast when you help them with a little bit of syringed colostrum during feeds. When you have risks for low supply, your breastfeeding plan might have to be different than the average blanket suggestions often regurgitated by many well-meaning professionals, friends, or family members.

Low Supply

Now that we have reviewed risk factors for low supply, I think we should review what low supply means exactly. It means you do not make enough milk for your baby to gain weight in appropriate amounts, and that need is different for every baby. In other words, it means supply output does not match baby's needed intake.

One person may make 20 ounces per day but have a baby that needs 30 ounces per day to gain weight well. A different baby that the same lactating person has later in life might be more petite and gain well with 20 ounces per day, so that person would have a full supply for that baby. The determination of low supply can be different with each breastfeeding relationship, and even change throughout the relationship. When a baby nurses after 1 year of age they need less milk so a parent that had low supply the first year may have enough to still go on to nurse past that first year and into toddlerhood.

True low supply is different from a perceived low supply because of the needs of the baby. A person may wish that they made 6 ounces per session, but they make 4, and their baby still does well. This person would have a perceived, and not true, low supply. There are many examples of perceived low supply, and if your supply is ever in question then you should be seeking an IBCLC.

Now, also consider what a person's capacity is to hold milk in each breast when it is most full. This is surprisingly not directly related to breast size, as most people assume. A breast might be full of mammary tissue and very little fat, having a small appearance. A breast might be full of fat but have very little mammary tissue, having a large appearance. A large breast does not guarantee a large capacity. This is shocking to most large breasted people who struggle with supply. When a large breast does match a large capacity, those people can store much more in one breast than any one baby would ever need at one feeding; I have seen one breast hold up to 20 ounces when full! Alternatively, in any size breast, it is possible that a person may only make 1 ounce in each breast to add up to 2 ounces per feed, and they must feed those 2 ounces every 2 hours to satisfy their baby. This would be 24 ounces per day and likely enough to grow well on for most babies. However, it would require nursing 12 times per 24 hours. A person might consider this a low supply if they are unable to keep up with the demands of this schedule, though technically they might be able to meet their baby's daily nutritional needs.

In general babies eat about 1 ounce per hour, sometimes smaller babies do well with a bit less and sometimes larger babies want a bit more. For a smaller baby 19-24 ounces might be a full supply, and that would be the lower limits of normal. For a larger baby they might want 5 ounce feeds 6 to 7 times per day, so 30-35 ounces would be a full supply for that baby, and that is probably the upper limit of normal. Just because a baby will take more than that, does not make it healthy or necessary. Weight gain, overall growth patterns, and properly meeting milestones are the important indicators of appropriate intake. Normal intake after 1 month of age can be anywhere from 2.5 to 5 ounces per feed with breastmilk, and babies eat 8-12 times per day the first few months. Sometimes babies eat less often, like 5-8 times per day, if they end up taking larger feeds. The amount they take is stable from 1 to 6 months until they start solids, and as they start gradually eating more solids this nutritional intake displaces milk intake.

I am going to go off topic here to compare breastmilk to formula, because this sabotages many breastfeeding people when they think they should be producing as much breastmilk as a formula fed baby eats. Formula babies eat larger quantities but less often, due to it digesting more slowly because it is harder to digest. The amount they need continues to increase because it is not a living substance that changes, like breastmilk. When babies get breast milk their intake is more constant, as their gut matures, they hold on to more of the milk. As the months go by, the proteins and other nutrition in the breastmilk also change to better suit the baby's needs. A formula fed baby might be taking 8 ounces per feed between 6-12 months, but a breastmilk fed baby should never do this. Occasionally, I see babies that want maybe 6 ounces per feed of breastmilk and do well with that, but most will stay in the 2.5 to 5-ounce range.

Returning to our topic of low supply, some good news is that most females grow more mammary tissue with each pregnancy. This means a person will most likely increase capacity with each pregnancy, and thus will likely make more milk after each pregnancy. However, if you have what is called insufficient glandular tissue, you will not likely increase mammary tissue dramatically enough with each pregnancy in order to have a full supply. This is because the glandular tissue did not develop enough in puberty, so the proper foundation of cells is not there.

There is also the chance that you have a great capacity but have some hormonal dysregulation, so your breasts are slow to refill with milk. Slow refill means the overall amount for the 24-hour period is insufficient, which can happen despite a normal capacity. An example might be pumping 3 ounces every 4 hours, which is only 18 ounces per 24 hours. The refill being slow would be indicated by still only getting 18 ounces daily even if you pump every 2 hours, getting 1.5 ounces per pump. The breast may have the capacity for 3 ounces, which can be a full feed for some babies, but if you are unable to get the 3 ounces often enough to get a daily total that is sufficient, then it is a slow refill. The refill adequacy is determined by the total of ounces per 24 hours, despite number of pump or nursing sessions changing.

While my examples are beautiful and simple math, most breasts do not work this way. The circadian rhythm of prolactin is such that it boosts from 12 to 5 AM and bottoms out in the early evening, and thus the milk supply is higher from midnight to noon than it is from noon to midnight. So, the breasts might make 4 to 5 ounces in the nighttime and early morning feeds but make only 2 to 3 ounces in the early evening feeds. The daily total is still the important number to look at.

All this leads us to needing to understand why low supply is important. Having enough milk intake is important to help your baby gain weight well. Why is weight gain so important? Generally, good weight gain indicates over-all growth that comes from the nutritional intake from breastmilk. Babies need to grow their skin, bones, muscles, and other organs more in complexity and size at an exponential rate the first few years of life. Not least of all, the brain does an immense amount of growing and developing in infancy. Babies need adequate nutrition in order to meet their milestones and develop optimally. In addition, the extra fat that they store is like an insurance plan for if they get sick, or you get sick, and they have a temporary reduction in food intake. The extra stored fat can be burned as energy when they are not eating well, protecting both the growth and the bodily functions, so that there is no interference due to the temporary circumstance.

It is also important because of the emotional impact on the person with low supply, and the clue that it provides that they may have a chronic underlying condition contributing to their low supply. Due to biological drive, the weight of not producing enough milk can feel like the weight of life and death. It can be emotionally and physically devastating, and exhausting. During pregnancy we are bombarded with "breast is best" mottos, without any real support or education behind them. Parents who experience supply struggles are significantly more at risk for postpartum mood disorders. Parents who have these struggles often take years to emotionally recover from the trauma. It is isolating because it is less common. It can be hard to reconcile the expectation of a full supply with the reality of a low supply. Parents often berate themselves and feel like failures. Sometimes the professionals that have failed these people shame and blame them, even though these parents have tried their hardest and done everything they know to do. Well-meaning friends and family might also insult their intelligence, or doubt that they have worked hard enough, or tried enough of the multitude of options available to try to improve supply. Even when they specifically say they do not want advice or have tried everything, people will still chime in. There is often an emotional struggle with negative emotions towards one's own breasts, and one's own body, one's own being. It can feel like they are robbed of an opportunity or a choice, which can feel an awful lot like being violated. It might feel like the body has betrayed them, because it has not delivered on an expectation. It might make them feel an ugly jealousy for those that it is going well for. It might conflict with intrinsic ideals of what a good parent should be. It can be deeply wounding to a mother's feelings of her identity as a woman, and as a parent. It can make one question if they were meant to be a mother. The hormones and biological drive involved in nursing make this feel fundamental to one's identity and goes deeper than logic. For many people with low supply, it transforms them. Few go through this and remain unchanged.

The handful of chronic underlying illnesses that can influence breast tissue development and milk supply regulation should be thoroughly assessed for in all lactating people with low supply. Too often it is brushed off and reduced to the explanation that "some women just can't breastfeed." No one should be being given this as a final answer, your healthcare providers should be seeking why it has happened, and all options to correct it. You may be faced with having to advocate for yourself if you are in this situation. There is currently no evidence-based diagnostic panel and treatment plan for females with lactation insufficiency. You can start with asking to be assessed for PCOS, thyroid dysregulation, insulin dysregulation, low prolactin, micronutrient deficiencies, and anemia. Compare your results to the optimal ranges for lactating people, and not the general population. As with any chronic health concern, you deserve a complete and thorough investigation into possible causes. You may be the only one on your healthcare team advocating for yourself.

Too many females are given the expectation that they will have no problem with supply as long as they work hard enough and make the right choices. Saying a parent is not working hard enough is a cruel and simplified way to lay all blame at their feet when it is likely they have never worked harder at anything in their life, and they are up against many things that they have no control over. We are bombarded from the time we are in-utero until our death with toxins and endocrine disrupters through our diet and lifestyle. Sometimes the influence of those makes it such that the breast never developed properly to begin with, or they leave the pituitary or thyroid below optimal functioning. Even those with a knowledgeable and wise support team sometimes cannot make a full supply due to assaults on their body from many years ago. People with chronic low supply are often not given the thorough medical support they need, even when there is a fixable problem, because there are simply not enough providers trained in lactation medicine. When they need a higher level of care, it is not available.

If you find yourself facing low supply, only you will be able to answer how much effort and how much milk is worth it to you. No one on your team or in your family can make the call to quit or should suggest you quit. The power of that decision lay entirely within you.

I find for most people it is reasonable to attempt to maximize their supply based on hormonal norms. For example, trying to bring in any milk after 2 to 3 weeks might be in vain, if your milk never increases beyond a few milliliters. After 2 to 3 weeks, we are no longer hormonally primed to bring milk in. If frequent pumping or nursing for several weeks did not induce the milk to "come in", then it is not going to. If you are able to get increasing amounts of milk the first 2 to 3 weeks, no matter how slow the increase, then you should be encouraged to keep trying. We are hormonally primed to keep boosting supply for the first 4 to 6 weeks after delivery. You can take many steps for the first

4 to 6 weeks to keep maximizing supply, and then settle into an easier long-term routine that helps protect the supply, and the nursing relationship if you are feeding directly at the breast. This might look like doing a breast, bottle, pump plan for the first month, and then cutting out pumping and switching over to just nursing and bottle feeding, or switching to just nursing with an SNS. A breast, bottle, pump plan means you do all three of those activities at each feeding session for most, if not all, sessions. This is a laborious and exhausting routine, and it is not meant to be done long term.

Some things to consider when contemplating how much breast milk matters to you are the content of the milk, the benefits for the female, and the benefits for the infant. As far as the content, there are millions of antibodies and other important substances in just 1 teaspoon of breastmilk that are not found in formula, so a full supply is not needed to confer the immunological and nutritional benefits. Also, babies are often happy to continue to nurse even with low supply when it is offered with or after some supplemental milk. They can have your milk for dessert instead of the main course, and you can both still get all the benefits of nursing. The benefits of nursing and lactation for a female and baby are largely determined by the length of time you nurse, lactate, or give breastmilk. The benefits are not "dose dependent," meaning a small amount can still provide all the benefits. It matters more that you nurse or provide breastmilk for a set amount of time, versus a set amount of ounces. See the "benefits of breastfeeding" section for more detail on that.

Another important aspect to consider is how low supply effects your relationship with your partner. Your partner may question if you are doing everything you can, or if you are trying to find a way out of breastfeeding. They might wound you by questioning your knowledge and your motivation. They might struggle with their own feelings of betrayal of unmet expectations. They will have their own ideas about breastfeeding importance, and their influence on your decisions will play a huge role in the struggles of breastfeeding.

Supply regulation, for millions of lactating people, is an ongoing struggle. It is not as rare as most people in the lactation community and the healthcare community assume. While less common than the billions of people with sufficient supply, there are still millions of people experiencing it. If the statistics are correct at a conservative estimation, which is arguable, then there are constantly millions of people struggling with milk supply at any given time. Just because this is a low number by comparison, that does not make it a rare occurrence. As rates of hormonal dysregulation illnesses rise in our modern society, so do the rates of low supply.

To a lesser extent, it may also impact your relationship with family or friends. Humans like to connect with other humans that are similar to them. We seek connection through shared experiences. So, family, friends, or acquaintances who are breastfeeding, or who breastfed in the past, might judge you or look down on you for not making enough milk. They will not grasp the lengths you have gone to in order to make breastfeeding work. You might have to take some space from friends and family that are not willing to listen or empathize. You might also need space from hearing about other people's abundant milk flow. While it is tempting to completely isolate, it will be important to seek connection with other low supply parents. There are many fruitful and compassionate low supply support groups, online and in person. It will be good for you to seek them out because hearing about shared experiences from others can be healing and validating.

It is unfair to put the entire burden of supply regulation on parents, knowing what we know about how common risk factors are, and how little support they receive versus how much they need. The current healthcare system, unfortunately, does put most of the burden on the parents to troubleshoot their own possible contributing factors to their chronic low supply. Support truly needs to be environmental, emotional, economical, logistical, cultural, and personal. We have a long way to go.

Pain and other problems with your breasts during breastfeeding

This is a big one. Will it hurt? It should generally not be painful to nurse if neither the female nor baby have underlying issues, once both have learned to breastfeed with good technique and baby is being brought to breast with as deep of a latch as possible. Few parents escape breast and nipple pain the first few weeks postpartum, because it is a time of practice and troubleshooting for both parent and baby.

Sometimes pain can be just an initial latch pain that resolves quickly and is likely related to positioning. However, a persistent latch pain throughout a feed can be from a shallow latch, oral dysfunction, flat or inverted nipples, vasospasm in the nipples, or oral tethers like tongue ties. Some nipple tenderness in the early weeks can be common and due to high estrogen from pregnancy lingering and keeping the nipples sensitive, and it can be from needing practice getting the baby on the breast with a deep latch and in comfortable positioning. No matter how many parents say breastfeeding is painful the first few weeks, that does not make it normal. Common does not mean normal. It just means breastfeeding people are not being adequately supported or educated.

Engorgement pain is something unrelated to techniques and is a normal physiological response to milk coming in. Engorgement is its own category of pain, and luckily temporary and relatively quick. Pain can also be a sign of infections like thrush or mastitis. Milk flow can also be blocked from clogs or blebs, which are painful, too. Additionally, when baby is teething sometimes the saliva changes and increased nursing frequency make the nipple tender, or baby might try to bite down seeking comfort on the gums. We will discuss all these potential pain sources in more detail.

A shallow latch means just what it sounds like! The breast tissue is not deep enough in the baby's mouth. The baby needs to take in areola and nipple, not just the nipple! Remember this is a new skill for you and your baby so it takes practice. Your lactation consultant should have some tricks up their sleeves to help with this. It is not a bad idea to look up some videos on getting a deep latch and practice this new skill with your hands and a baby doll to start developing some muscle memory. You can play around with different positions and holds to see what feels most comfortable to you, so when you have a screaming baby ready to eat you are not scrambling and guessing which one you like best. Some examples you can look up are cross-cradle, cradle, football, laid-back, and side-lying. Keep in mind your favorite might not be the baby's favorite, so try to get comfortable with a few different positions so that you have options.
When latching try to avoid pushing on your baby's head to bring him to the breast. They have an anti-smother reflex that will cause them to pull back and get angry if you do this. It is best to gently push them from the shoulders to bring them towards the breast. This will allow their head to fall back, their chin to lift and come forward first, and enable a happier baby and deeper latch.

Flat or inverted nipples can cause difficulty or pain when you start nursing, as well. This makes it harder for babies to latch, but not impossible. The nipple is sort of stuck in that position and when the baby or the pump pulls the nipple out it breaks the adhesions on the skin that keep it stuck. The adhesions are similar to the ones that keep your nails on your nail beds. As you can imagine, breaking those adhesions is painful. Eventually, for most people, that stops hurting as the body learns to not keep re-attaching those tissues.

Nipple size plays a role in comfort as well. Large nipples

may pose a challenge if they are large enough to stop the baby from being able to fit it in their mouth. Additionally, the tissue behind the nipple needs to be elastic to mold deeply into the baby's mouth, so a more firm or fibrous breast may present some challenges with obtaining a deep latch.

In the early nursing days, nipple tenderness and engorgement are largely hormonal. Note that sore and tender is normal while intense pain and nipple damage is not. Estrogen is a big player in nipple soreness and tenderness. It is high when you are pregnant due to the placenta and the endometrial lining build up, so things should calm down after a few weeks postpartum as estrogen drops. The nipple sensitivity decreases as time goes on because of the diminished estrogenic effect, and many people incorrectly call this the nipples "toughening up" as they assume the process is attributed to the nipple skin callousing or becoming thicker.

When your milk comes in, typically day 3 to 5 postpartum, most experience the engorgement pain I keep mentioning. The body responds to this change by basically panicking and sending water around the mammary tissues as an immune system response. This also often accompanies a huge hormonal surge that makes you cry frequently. As the tears flow, the milk flows. You also have extra water swelling throughout the whole body from retained extra fluid during pregnancy. That fluid shifting around and trying to leave the body is what causes the general swelling. The fluid in your arms and legs will often shift down to your feet, as gravity pulls it down. The extreme fullness, and the skin being tight as a result, causes pain. The pain resolves relatively quickly, in a day or two. The swelling may linger for a few weeks, as the shedding of extra fluid has to be a slow process in order to protect your electrolyte balance. Massage, frequent nursing, ice packs, elevating your feet, and ibuprofen will be your friends!

Initially, your nipples may get damaged which will cause pain. Cracks, bleeding, scabs, bruises, and blisters are actually pretty common. Remember, common does not mean normal.

We need a baby to be latching and removing milk without damaging the nipple. This initial damage is usually due to lack of practice with getting a deep latch, and the difficulty of getting a deep latch when you are engorged. Ongoing pain might result from the nipple being re-injured repeatedly or not being given a chance to heal with a break from latching. Sometimes the injury is related to muscle tension or poor coordination of the oral muscles in the baby. The good news is, if there are no oral tethers in the baby's mouth then it should heal quickly, within days, even with re-latching 8-12 times per day. Oral dysfunction and oral tethers will be covered under the "Your Baby" chapter. Once the latch is corrected, it should not continue to re-injure the nipple. A lactation consultant can help you learn to latch the baby deeply and position to comfort. This can even be practiced, to an extent, before baby is born. They can also help you with tips for allowing the nipples to heal if they do get damaged, while still protecting your supply.

Another source of pain can be a yeast infection, called thrush. Thrush is an infection that can be on your nipples and in your baby's mouth. It is actually what we call an "opportunistic" infection. Yeast that live on your skin and in your digestive tract take the opportunity to multiply when conditions are favorable. The yeast can thrive when bacterial counts are low, and the conditions are dark and moist. Yeast lives on and in our bodies and can also cause vaginal yeast infection, jock itch, and foot fungus! The symptoms are similar no matter the body part; itching, pink skin, and pain! On the nipples it can be very bright pink and there will be stabbing, burning, shooting pains. These can be felt on the nipples, as well as within the ducts in the breast. In the baby's mouth it can look like round white patches. Those who are old enough to talk usually say oral thrush causes some pain and tenderness in the oral cavity and throat. A bacterial infection may also be present, especially if the infections are associated with breaks in the skin. Seek a professional for assessment and to determine appropriate treatment, to be sure. Other than an appropriate medication, you will need help identifying the cause of infection and a plan to prevent it from reoccurring.

It is also important to note that not every provider is currently practicing the most evidence-based care of thrush in a breastfeeding dyad. If either you or your baby is diagnosed, you both must be treated. This is because the yeast count needs to be lowered in both of you in order for one or both of you to re-balance and heal. This will make choosing who to see for thrush tricky. If you seek thrush treatment for your baby, the pediatrician cannot prescribe you treatment. If you go to your obstetrician for nipple thrush treatment, they will not prescribe for your baby. It is best to seek treatment for both of you, and that includes sterilizing everything that touches your nipples or your baby's mouth. Even pumping parents get thrush, and this advice applies to them as well. You will need to involve an IBCLC to get the most thorough treatment plan for your specific circumstances; even better if the IBCLC is also a family or midwife provider because they can then prescribe for you and the baby.

Clogged ducts, blebs and mastitis are other causes of breast and nipple pain. The duct is like the hallway that the milk flows down. Clogged ducts might be referred to as clogs, blocked ducts, or lumps. They are typically felt just under the skin as a small circular or oval firm area that is tender to the touch. They are often accompanied by some pink, redness, and bruising over the clogged area. They can occur anywhere along the milk line, but are typically in the breast, and they can be very painful. Clogs or swelling occurs for many females in the axilla region during engorgement, this can be an area where the milk comes in because there is mammary tissue, but has nowhere to flow out of because there is no nipple and no ducts connect to it. If you use ice and compression it will resolve in a few days. Blocked ducts can occur in the breast when milk is not removed frequently enough, the milk is not drained thoroughly, baby has a poor latch, one is using poorly fitting pump flanges, or one has a milk bleb that is blocking flow. Some people describe them as feeling like beans or peas under the skin, and they are usually tender and sore. If the opportunistic bacteria in the ducts start over-growing or the immune system starts to attack the clog, then you are going to get symptoms of an infection called mastitis. The symptoms will be a large area of redness over the skin, the breast being hot to touch, breast and body pain, fevers, chills, and feeling generally ill or weak. Antibiotics will be needed from a provider if you have a fever over 100.4 degrees Fahrenheit (38 degrees Celsius) or several of these symptoms. Even more importantly, you have to release that clog! If you do not get the milk flowing, the clog can abscess, which would require surgical drainage and packing. You will not only need heat and massage to increase flow, but you will also need ice and medicine to decrease inflammation. See an IBCLC to help make a treatment plan, because it will depend on what is causing the clogging. You will not only want to treat the current clog, but also prevent future clogs. If frequent clogging is an issue you can discuss with your IBCLC if you are a good candidate for sunflower lecithin, in addition to troubleshooting the source of the clogging.

Next, we discuss a nipple injury known as milk blebs or milk blisters. They are little fluid filled sacks on the tip of the nipple, cause by friction. Usually caused by a poor pump flange fit, a bad latch, or both. Blebs block the flow out of the ducts and thus can lead to clogs, and thus mastitis. On their own they are extremely painful. A lactation consultant can help you make a plan to clear those clogs and release those blebs, and there are several helpful tips to try first available online. Just like with clogs, getting the milk flowing is the immediate priority and you will want to evaluate how to prevent getting more of them, which a professional might help with.

Other possible problems in the breasts are an overactive letdown and an oversupply. It sounds like a lovely problem to have too much milk, but notice I still called it a "problem?" That is because it can cause severe gastrointestinal discomfort for your baby, cause your baby to reject the breast, cause pain from frequently overly full breasts, make you more prone to clogs and mastitis, and make your life revolve around pumping frequently to relieve your pain and prevent some of these issues.

Oversupply also causes babies to get too much foremilk and not get enough fatty hindmilk, and at times the strong flow overwhelms them. They are often eating excessively frequently, having mucous in the stool, excessive gas, stomach discomfort, and excessive weight gain. For families it can cause logistical issues with food storage in the fridge and freezer, often creating a need for an extraneous expense of buying an extra freezer. Freezing your bags flat can help save space, and you can always donate extra that you cannot accommodate for, so space might not be a problem. It can be hard to correct an oversupply without over-correcting, and then not having enough milk. It can be a long and tedious process to correct over-supply. You will likely want to make sure you avoid over stimulating the milk production in the early weeks postpartum to avoid these problems.

Another common issue with oversupply is the guilt or inner turmoil parents face with stopping breastfeeding when it is affecting their mental health or physical health. When you have an abundant supply you might be plagued with thoughts around how it is selfish or unjust of you to take this gift away from your baby when you produce it so easily. Stopping or reducing pumping, or switching to formula can be a very hard choice to make.

Most parents can avoid over supply if they pump minimally for convenience or comfort, and only frequently if they are supplementing. Many lactating people pump themselves into an over-supply because they know they need to drain their breasts every feeding, but they are not trusting that their baby is doing that, so they follow up breastfeeding with pumping. Many also pump to drain when they should only be pumping to relieve. The main goals should be to allow your baby to regulate your supply to their needs. If you over-pump you will encourage an over-supply. You should only be following a breastfeeding and pumping routine if you are supplementing, and it is meant to be short term and temporary. If you are unsure if you should be pumping, that is when you should seek professional help. The initial engorgement period is typically when over-pumping starts for most over-suppliers.

Alternatively, some people have a hyperlactation syndrome where they make too much milk from the beginning despite not overstimulating, and they should be working with an IBCLC as soon as possible to help discourage the oversupply as much as possible. If you suspect you have an over-supply and it is causing issues for you and/or your baby, make an appointment as soon as you are able.

There is also of course the consideration that some people desire an oversupply. Parents might wish to be ahead of their own child's needs, want to donate breastmilk to babies in need, or sell their milk. Some people also just enjoy the sorting, storing, and counting aspects of pumping and end up with an oversupply and extra milk stash due to that.

There are a few donation services that will pay you for your labor and help replace parts and bags. Most donation centers expect a free and clear donation and have strict screening processes; they will test you for diseases and want to know all medications and herbs you take and will have you on a strict protocol for sanitizing your parts and storing your milk properly. Most donated milk goes to the most medically fragile infants who are in the hospital, but parents can also buy it from you or donation centers after they are at home. The donation centers are non-profit but have to charge for the milk in order to pay for the testing and pasteurization of the milk, and the labor of the staff.

Parents of older infants also seek donations when they are unable to make enough milk and are usually happy to replace your bags and pumping supplies, as needed. Peer to peer donation is usually built around avoiding monetary exchange to avoid temptation to water down or add cow milk to the breast milk bags. Parents will often ask for medical records proving you have no diseases that can pass through breast milk, and want to know about your diet, lifestyle, and medications. Many strong bonds and friendships can come from the exchange of milk-sharing, and parents are usually very grateful. In some cultures, sharing milk makes babies "milk-siblings" and they cannot ever be married. I find this old practice especially interesting, because now we know that breastmilk stem cells go on to become part of the baby's body, and so taking on another person's milk makes them part of you.

Body builders and other adults are often also interested in purchasing of extra milk. If you decide to encourage over supply in order to sell or donate milk then it should be from an informed space, knowing the possible risks. I would encourage work with an IBCLC for that as well, to help minimize risks.

People with oversupply often also have and overactive letdown, because of the overfullness of the breasts causing more pressure buildup, but it is possible to have one without the other. An overactive letdown is when your letdown is too forceful for the baby to handle. They often experience choking, gagging, pulling away from the breast, excessive gas, mucous in the stools, difficulty with feeling satisfied, and sometimes breast refusal. Alternative positioning and other strategies can often help in these situations.

Leaking of milk when not feeding is a problem often erroneously associated with oversupply, but many with a low or regular supply leak as well. Milk leaking from the nipple is based on how tight and strong the muscles are behind the nipple, and unfortunately you cannot exercise those particular muscles. Biologically, milk being able to flow easily is beneficial to the survival of babies—especially those struggling to pull the milk out. While flowing easily can be advantageous to more easily feeding babies, it can also be messy! Leaking or unexpected letdowns can be triggered by many things, crying babies, the smell of baby products, emotional upset, and even orgasms. Some people are sad to find out that they still cannot sleep on their stomach after the baby comes, because it causes leaking. Most people work around leaking by using breast pads, milk catchers, and towels. Milk catchers and silicone suction devices are a handy way to easily build an extra stash, because if you are going to leak you might as well save that milk. Leaking may stop after a few months, and this does not automatically mean you have stopped making enough milk. Having a change of clothes for you in the diaper bag or pumping bag is also helpful if you might leak through your clothes. Honestly, that is helpful to have anyway because you never know when your baby will poop or vomit all over your outfit.

The let-down or ejection reflex itself can be painful, itchy, or induce negative emotions. The let-down is when the hormones from the brain travel down to the breast which causes the milk to flow down the ducts and out of the nipple to the baby in gushes or spurts. It causes the muscles around the ducts to squeeze the milk out. When this is a new or unfamiliar sensation and the brain does not recognize how to interpret it, sometimes it can misfire and categorize it as pain or itching. The pain also might be related to the intensity of the hormonal response. Some describe the sensation as glass shards, intense itching, pins and needles, tickling, or a thick course yarn being pulled through the breast towards the nipple. This usually subsides after a few weeks as the breasts get used to it and the intensity of the hormones diminishes.

The let-down hormones causing negative emotions is called DMER--Dysphoric Milk Ejection Reflex. In most females the release of the hormone oxytocin that occurs during let-down elicits feelings of pleasure. Dysphoric is a fancy way of saying that it does not illicit feelings of pleasure, as expected, but rather unpleasant feelings. For people that experience DMER let-downs can bring up many negative emotions like panic, sadness, anger, irritability, or grief. It can produce physical responses like nausea, muscle tension, or hot flashes. It is usually most intense the first few weeks postpartum and can be so intense it leads some people to choose to wean. If you push through it, it is a limited and temporary response that does eventually get better. Sometimes just knowing what it is, that it is temporary, and that you are not alone is enough to keep you going! For many people, it makes them dread nursing and feel guilty about not enjoying it.

Sometimes the nursing aversion is not related to the letdown, and some people just experience negative feelings the entire time baby is latched. Sometimes this is avoided or reduced by pumping. Feelings might be similar to DMER, such as irritability, anger, agitation, restlessness, skin-crawling, self-loathing, and dread.

Letdown can also be weak and slow, especially with low supply, but not always. Smoking, caffeine intake, and alcohol consumption can be contributing factors. Any risks for low supply also present as risks for a weak letdown. Reassuringly, you do not need to have a very fast letdown, it just needs to be fast enough to keep the baby interested.

Vasospasms in the nipples or ducts are also something that can be painful when breastfeeding, which may or may not happen with letdown. Vasospasm is when the vascular flow is restricted suddenly, and the body part experiencing the spasm turns white from lack of blood flow, and it is very painful. People with Raynaud's Syndrome or other similar conditions often experience this phenomenon right after a nursing session. It is often misdiagnosed as thrush because of the shooting sensations sometimes felt, and this is also a common thrush symptom. There is medication your healthcare provider can trial with you if this is too intense of a problem. For most people it resolves or starts to dramatically diminish after the first 4-6 weeks of nursing.

Pain associated with breastfeeding is not always found in the breast. Sometimes the pain is elsewhere in the body, such as at a surgical incision site that hurts due to positioning, following a cesarean delivery or tubal ligation. There is often painful trapped gas that keeps you from being able to achieve or stay in optimal positioning, as it creates an urgency to move to try to get the trapped air out. Surgery causes us to have to get creative with breastfeeding positioning to avoid putting pressure on the incision site with the weight of the baby's body. Sometimes the pain is musculoskeletal because of hormonal changes, as well as new positions and muscle strains. This can give parents symptoms similar to arthritis and carpal tunnel when pregnant and nursing.

Next, we will go over milk color changes. This can be confusing and alarming to many parents, but it is not actually a problem in most cases. Fun Fact: Your milk is not always white! It is first a golden yellow when it is colostrum in the end of pregnancy and the early days of nursing. It typically slowly adjusts to white within 3 to 5 days postpartum. However, it can be many colors, usually based on your diet. A big batch of blueberries might tint it blue! Eat a lot of greens? Guess what? Green tinted milk! If it is pink it is likely from a bit of blood from an injury on your nipple, or a harmless growth in the breast, and is safe to feed. If it comes out of the breast white but then turns red after being out a while, this might be a harmful bacteria over-populating. It is never wrong when in doubt to seek professional guidance on if your milk is safe to feed or not.

The other perceived issue when looking at pumped milk is the fat content you are able to visualize. Sometimes, some of the fat separates out and gels at the top of the bottle, which looks like a large fat plug. Even if yours does not do this, there is likely still plenty of fat in it. The fat amount varies throughout the day and is generally higher in a more drained breast so more frequent feedings usually have higher fat content. You can eat more healthy fats to help improve the ratios of types of fats in the milk, but it is unlikely to increase the fat content. Your baby needs the higher water volume of foremilk for hydration, and the higher concentration of fatty globules in the hindmilk for growth. Trust that your milk is made perfectly, the body has tens of thousands of years of practice built into its genetic coding. If you pump a large amount in one sitting be sure to mix it all together before separating it for feeds to ensure there is foremilk and hindmilk in each bottle.

Morning milk tends to have more volume, and less fat. Babies need to hydrate in the morning after going long stretches without drinking. Night milk tends to have less volume but more fat, and the higher fat in a full belly allows for greater satiety and longer stretches between feeds. Depending on the time of day the milk will have different levels of hormones and other particles to encourage baby to be awake or to sleep, such as melatonin. It is available in the milk to work with baby's natural hormone rhythms to encourage sleep and wake cycles, it is not enough to over-power the patterns so do not worry too much about keeping track of what time you pumped your milk. Parents who do not track time pumped versus time fed have not reported a higher incidence of sleep issues in their infants. It does not hurt to track this and try to match these up, especially if you are struggling with getting to a normal sleep and wake pattern. It is not something to obsess over, just keep an eye on.

Pumped milk can also reveal a problem of having high lipase. Lipase is what helps break down the fats in the milk, and when there is a lot of it in pumped milk it can alter the smell and flavor. It can cause some babies to refuse pumped milk. It might taste or smell rancid, soapy, or metallic. It might change after a few hours, or only change after it has been frozen. This is easily remedied by scalding the milk right after it is pumped, which kills off some of the lipase. You would do well to test if you have high lipase before you start building a freezer stash in case you have a baby that refuses it.

Pumped milk also inevitably begs the question of how it is different from fresh milk. Fresh milk is dynamic and changes to fit the baby's needs. Frozen milk may smell or taste different and have less white blood cells, less protein, less Vitamin C, and less antibacterial properties. It is still superior to donor milk or formula, when from the biological parent of the infant.

Additionally, a perceived problem many females have is the lack of symmetry in their breasts. This includes size, capacity, flow rate, and nipple size. Few things in nature are perfectly symmetrical. It helps to think of the breasts as sisters and not twins. Often one breast produces 3 to 5 times as much milk as the other. Some parents even successfully nurse on one breast only. The letdown on one side might come more easily or come out faster. Nipples are often different sizes on each breast. The ways in which one breast differs from the other can be multiple things. These are not problems that need fixing, just natural variations.

Challenges within the parent

Finally, we go over parental sided problems not of the breasts but of the mind; self-sabotage, self-doubt, and self-criticism. We can often be our own worst enemy and our own worst critics. This is especially true when the stakes are high, there is high emotional attachment, and especially with breastfeeding, where our ego and our maternal identity is tied into our perception of succeeding.

Parents often will sabotage their own breastfeeding relationship by frequently topping off a baby with pumped milk or formula. They do this when the baby is rooting frequently or seems unsatisfied after eating. Frequent rooting and seeming to not be satisfied after some feeds are innate and instinctive behaviors that serve several biological purposes. It is unrelated to how nourished or hydrated the baby is, unless you have verified that the baby is not gaining weight well, you can attribute it to normal behavior. Babies are designed to cluster feed and act unsatisfied in order to call your body to boost supply the first 4 to 6 weeks of life. Frequent nursing also forces you to sit still and rest at a time that you need to be; when you are recovering from pregnancy and delivery. They also nurse frequently when they have growth spurts. When you interrupt this pattern with top-off bottles you miss critical signaling to the body to keep boosting supply. Frequent feeding also serves to help keep babies alive and well cared for when they regularly wake and request your attention. If you want to know that your baby is getting enough milk then you need to monitor the diaper count daily and the weight gain every few days in the first two weeks, and then weekly in the first 6 weeks. Even weekly can be excessive when things are understood to be going well.

It is too easy to criticize ourselves and falsely equalize breastfeeding success and ease with parenting ability and parenting success. This is especially hard for people with anxious tendencies. It is even harder when you compare yourself to other parents and you perceive that their journey was easy without knowing the whole story. Modern parents often push themselves too hard and blame themselves for things outside of their control. Do not buy into those lies! Turn off those negative thoughts. Breastfeeding is hard and challenging; that is why there is an entire profession that exists to help troubleshoot it!

Self-sabotage and self-doubt also happen often with milestones, and especially when we start babies on solids. This begins the process of "weaning," slowly adding solids that eventually replace the milk as the main nutrition source. If you feed baby solids first then offer the breast, they will start to take more solids than breastmilk, and this is undesirable the first year. Between 6 to 12 months when you offer solids it is ideal to breastfeed first, then offer the solids. After 1 year of age you can do either sequence. It can be a helpful tool to either help discourage or encourage nursing frequency, depending on your goals. If you have food allergies you might want to rinse your baby's mouth before latching to the breast to avoid skin irritation, while still allowing them the exposure to the food to reduce their chance of developing allergies.

If your self-criticism and self-doubt is interfering with your ability to get things accomplished or move forward with goals or plans, then it is time to seek help. You can start building self-trust through several helpful practices. Practicing mindfulness can help you to identify your emotions and be more in-touch with the present reality and take you away from your negative thought process. Journaling patterns can help you get to the root of where this negative internal feedback stems from and can help you differentiate it from the truth. You can also give yourself internal validation with positive self-talk and affirmations or leave yourself notes with those mantras all over your house. The more you hear them the more ingrained they become. Try to quiet the outside voices from external critics and focus on the facts. If these steps are not enough, it might be time for counseling.

Some final thoughts I have about what is hard and challenging from the parent's perspective are around the other psychological challenges. For example, how hard it can be to sit and nurse for so many hours a day. When we have our first baby it can come as quite a shock how much we have to sit and be still. When we are accustomed to being able to hop up and do things at-will it is ridiculously hard to relinquish our control to our baby's whims. Most of us sit and contemplate all the things we could be getting done. In these moments it helps to remind yourself that you are in fact getting something done. You are feeding your baby and meeting their needs for comfort and closeness. In the early weeks this will also promote the rest that your body needs in order to heal.

Additionally, many people find they are having to learn to ask for and accept help where they have not had to routinely do this for many years. Making peace with the modern expectation placed on parents being unrealistic can help you open up to knowing that needing help at this time is actually normal and expected. It is unrealistic to expect a parent to juggle as much as we ask them to while recovering, and healing, and changing. Start building your village before the baby comes and get comfortable with reaching out, even if it feels awkward do it anyway! Your mental health depends on it.

Your heart will grow in ways you did not know it could, and while for some people that feels good, it can also make adults who were neglected or abused as children extremely uncomfortable. The big feelings and the big love can be heartbreaking as you reflect on what you missed out on, and at the same time also be very healing to know this kind of love and connection is possible between parent and child. It can be a time of many conflicting emotions, and growth.

Finally, I want you to be prepared to grieve. Even when looking forward to the changes that parenthood brings many people find they grieve for the person they once were and the life they once had. This does not make you a bad parent, it makes you a normal human. When we transition to new roles in life, we go through this. You might remember grieving childhood as you stepped into adolescence, yet you still enjoyed the growth and the freedom that it brought you. You can still be a good parent and enjoy being a parent, while also being disappointed with it and grieving for what was.

The Baby

Even when you have a healthy full-term infant with no complications during pregnancy and labor, having a new baby can feel like you moved to a new country and you do not speak the language. The learning curve is steep. Additionally, no one wants to hear this, and no one wants to approach the subject, but not all babies are born full term or without health conditions. Your baby might face challenges like being smaller than average (usually called small for gestational age or SGA), being born premature, get a birth injury, or have a health condition. Most of these things interfere with breastfeeding ability and efficiency. Even a slightly early but "full term" 37-week gestational age baby is at risk for not being an efficient feeder. In breastfeeding, a generally healthy baby is not all that matters.

Some health conditions prevent babies from draining the breast well because they get tired, like some heart or lung conditions. Some conditions increase caloric demand, like reflux, cystic fibrosis, or heart conditions. Sometimes there is temporary neuromuscular damage that influences feeding efficiency, such as injury during delivery with shoulder dystocia or vacuum use. Sensory processing disorders and poor or high muscle tone can also influence the breastfeeding relationship. Some structural anomalies or muscular abnormalities can also prevent the baby from moving their mouth and tongue as needed to get the milk to flow and to efficiently drain the breast. Even still, sometimes babies have unexplained poor tone and oral motor function. Your baby might need to work with the speech and language pathology team, as they often handle feeding difficulties through occupational and physical therapies.

Listing all the possible ways the health of the infant might influence feeding is actually not going to be exhaustively covered in this book, so keep in mind if your baby is diagnosed in utero or as a newborn with any health conditions it will be an important question to ask how it might influence breastfeeding. This question really should be asked of every member of your healthcare team, which should include an IBCLC. Most babies, no matter the challenge, should be given the chance to breastfeed.

We will explore some of the most common challenges with babies in the breastfeeding relationship in more detail here.

Prematurity or SGA

Babies are born premature for many reasons and if yours is you can expect breastfeeding to be challenging, but not impossible. Many full-term infants who are small for gestational age (SGA) tend to struggle with breastfeeding as well, and in many ways behave like a premature infant. Premature babies need more help because of neurological and muscular immaturity. They do not have the needed reflexes, strength, and coordination in order to suckle, swallow, and breathe in a nice efficient pattern; nor to maintain that activity long enough to get sufficient amounts of milk before tiring out. Premature and SGA babies often have to ease into breastfeeding over several months while they develop neurological maturity, strength, and coordination.

The parent of a premature infant needs more support because they have missed the last one to three months of breast tissue development, and they are often separated from their infant and missing out on crucial biological cues in order to bring in and increase milk supply. When a lactating parent-infant dyad is separated they do not get as much skin to skin, they cannot smell each other, and the baby is not near-constantly suckling to bring more milk in. Females need to feel baby's warm body, smell their scents, hear their crying, and have them at the breast frequently in order for the body to know the infant has survived and needs feeding. This is biological and needs to be addressed with every dyad separated by a NICU (Neonatal Intensive Care Unit) stay, not just premature infants. The loss of those exchanges between parent and infant will need replicated and replaced as much and as closely as possible, and the parent needs to be able to visit and hold baby as much as possible.

We have a term called "late preterm" to describe babies who are 34-36 weeks gestation. They are the most stable and most developed of premature infants, but they are still immature in many systems and developmental milestones. The experience with a 28-week premature infant is very different than a 36-week premature infant. A NICU stay for a late preterm infant may not even occur, or be weeks to months shorter than the stay for preterm infants born between 23 to 34 weeks. Each week in utero baby gains more strength, coordination, and additional reflexes; all important to feeding. All infants born 37 weeks gestation or younger are considered higher risk for feeding difficulties, as well as other health conditions. It is crucial that even after discharge from the hospital, you maintain close and frequent contact with their healthcare team, including your IBCLC.

If your child is premature in addition to working with a lactation consultant, you will likely need a healthcare team to get your baby feeding and growing optimally. Premature infants often need their breastmilk fortified to increase the calories and decrease the workload of eating. Fortifiers are usually made from formula, but human milk fortifiers are becoming more available. If your child has health conditions that require intervention the team might be even bigger and more complex. The team might include a nutrition specialist, feeding specialist, speech and language pathologist, occupational and physical therapy, gastrointestinal specialist, and other specialists or surgeons depending on your child's specific needs. Covering all of those health possibilities is outside the scope of this book, just know that help is available!

Birth Injuries and Temporary Musculoskeletal Issues

Sometimes during labor and delivery the infant can sustain an injury, or the way baby is positioned in utero and in labor can cause muscle strain. Examples of birth injuries are when the baby has a broken clavicle, a bruised head, muscle strain in the neck or jaw, excessive head molding, or a bruised face. Birth injuries are possible with spontaneous vaginal deliveries that have minimal to no intervention, so there is always a risk of occurrence. Even being positioned certain ways in the last few weeks in the womb can result in head, jaw, and neck tension in the baby. Any of these conditions might influence the tone, coordination, comfort, and efficiency of breastfeeding. Babies might need some infant massage or other body work if this is the case. It just might take them a longer time than usual to really become efficient and pain free at the breast. Sometimes a one-sided tension expresses as one-sided pain with latching. All these conditions might necessitate some extra work for a few days, or a few weeks, while baby adjusts and heals. This might be something your pediatrician or lactation consultant points out. There is often a need for pumping and/or supplementing in addition to some body work. Depending on the birth injury, you will need a personalized plan from your healthcare team, including the IBCLC, to determine the best positions to feed, tools that might be helpful, or just how much need there is to adjust the feeding to accommodate the baby.

Some temporary and transitional conditions require that baby be supplemented, for example while waiting for your milk to come in your baby might lose too much weight or become dehydrated. This does not always happen, but several studies show that it happens to a majority of first-time parents, so it is worth mentioning. Supplementation during this time can be so that they do not become dehydrated, too jaundiced, or have too low of blood sugars. If you do not pump during this temporary supplementation then you are missing critical stimulation because the baby is not going to the breast as much, if at all. Your brain must be stimulated via suckling frequently at the breast to know biologically that an infant has survived and needs feeding. The pump will act as the suckling babe in these cases. If you desire to breastfeed and need to supplement, then in order to not risk your long-term supply you must pump every time supplementation is offered.

What needs to be more normalized is the expectation of supplementing your baby the first week of life, especially for first time parents. To pretend it is unlikely for first-time parents sets us up for emotional turmoil and emotional upset. For tens of thousands of years, we have relied on other lactating people and other animals to help us provide milk for our babies until our milk came in. Almost half of females having their first child experience their milk coming in later than the expected 3-5 days. Statistically, most of these families benefit from a temporary supplementation plan because it relieves stress and pressure around caring for the infant and helps ensure the infant is healthy and stable. Supplementation can be a parent's pumped or hand expressed milk, donor milk, or formula. Studies have shown that carefully monitored minimal supplementation during the first week actually leads to better long-term success with establishing and maintaining breastfeeding, because it helps get baby off to a good physical start and helps parents have reduced stress around the process. Babies need to be well hydrated and have enough nutritional intake to be able to nurse well, so if that is not happening things can go very poorly within just a few days. This is why close follow up is suggested the first week or two postpartum. The key is not to supplement without also providing extra stimulation to the breast, which is done with hand expression and pumping.

Some conditions can sometimes make baby so fragile that they have to temporarily be separated from you to go to the NICU, or in jaundice cases be inside a special blanket with lights or a special bed with lights. You might get a lot of push-back or pushing-around from nurses and doctors who are accustomed to freely giving formula when you approach options other than formula to address these concerns. To them formula is part of a safe, easy, and effective treatment plan. They come from a logical place of wanting to keep your baby safe through using the formula in a medicinal way. This can clash with a strong emotional desire to only provide breast milk. Remember, even the World Health Organization and other leading health agencies say that formula is great when there is a medical need. Medical needs include jaundice, low blood sugar, and dehydration. If you do not have enough breast milk or donor milk, then formula is the next best and safest option whenever not supplementing is not an option.

Jaundice is a common reason to need to supplement. Jaundice is caused by the build-up of bilirubin, the byproduct of red blood cell breakdown. The baby breaks down a large number of red blood cells after birth. Every baby goes through this process, and some studies suggest the build-up of the bilirubin might be protective against sepsis. What we watch for is the number or build-up of the bilirubin to not get too high. Our liver is what breaks the bilirubin down, and then dumps it into our bowels and urine so we can poop and urinate it out of our bodies. Giving more milk helps the body break down and flush out the bilirubin through the bladder and bowels. If needed, the special blankets help break the bilirubin down, reducing the workload on the liver. Jaundice does not absolutely require formula, as pumped or donor milk can help, and light therapy might be the only extra treatment needed. There is nothing magical in formula that helps fight jaundice, rather, it is the increase in volume intake that helps flush out the jaundice. If there is not enough volume of pumped or donor milk, formula is the next best option.

Breastfeeding jaundice and breast milk jaundice are often confused. Breastfeeding jaundice is often from not enough volume of milk to help pass the bilirubin out of the body; this usually develops in the first week of life. If you increase the baby's intake it should help, whether that is pumped milk or formula. When a baby develops enough jaundice for the medical team to be concerned and suggest intervention it is also often when the breastfeeding relationship becomes threatened. This is a great time to ask questions like the following:

- Can we supplement with pumped milk for 24 hours and re-evaluate?
- Can we do the light therapy and continue with breastmilk and then re-evaluate?
- Have we included a lactation consultant in this treatment and feeding plan?

Breast milk jaundice sounds terribly similar but is different. It is a phenomenon of breastfed babies tending to be jaundiced several weeks longer than formula fed babies, it also usually develops later than day 7. The longer time period is not dangerous, and we are not entirely sure why it happens. Sometimes a break from breastfeeding is needed to drop the levels if they are dangerously high, but then breastfeeding can be resumed.

Jaundice can be physiological (typical and expected like those just mentioned) or pathological (resulting from disease in the body). Pathological jaundice appears within the first 24 hours, rather than 2-3 days into breastfeeding, because it is related to something happening in the baby's body rather than as a result of breastfeeding issues. In extreme cases the baby might need a blood transfusion, intravenous medications, or additional tests to rule out underlying diseases, in addition to the supplemental feeding and light therapies typically used.

While waiting for your milk to come in is not necessarily a medical need for supplementation itself, supplementing can prevent some medical issues from arising during that time. Many parents are comfortable with and happy to supplement minimally while waiting for the milk to start to flow in larger volumes. Your healthcare team is watching for signs that the baby might need supplemented, because scary things can happen if we miss the cues. When a baby does not get enough milk their blood sugar can drop, and if it drops low enough it can lead to seizures. The baby may become dehydrated, which is a threat to their life. It may feel sometimes like supplementation is pushed because healthcare providers do not want to risk these things happening when it is safe to supplement. Other than those physical needs it might also meet the needs of the parents to feel reassured about how well their baby is being fed. It can also take some of the pressure off of the lactating parent. Babies who are well hydrated and have good energy levels after a little bit of supplementation will often do better at the breast. There is research and anecdotal evidence that early and minimal supplementation in conjunction with lactation support actually helps parents meet their long-term breastfeeding goals.

While it is likely true that milk has taken 3 to 5 days to come in since the beginning of human existence, it is also true that our lifestyles are vastly different. In days past we used to have several lactating people physically close to us that would nurse our babies until our milk came in, or we would borrow from the family goat. We are a resilient species, and part of the reason for that is our flexibility in our diet. I think we need to keep that in mind.

Today, we have formula and donor milk, rather than close relatives or family cows. It is also best to look at formula in some of these cases as a medical intervention. It will keep your baby alive and well, and does not mean that you will not still meet your breastfeeding goals. If the idea of formula is being brought up and you are planning to breastfeed then a lactation consultant needs to be on the healthcare team that is making plans and decisions. You will need to follow a plan that you make with a lactation consultant to bring in your milk and protect your supply.

If donor milk might be an option for your baby, you will want to talk to your partner about it. Some people find they prefer formula to donor milk, or vice versa. It is important to sit and think about your feelings around which supplemental milk to use when you are calm and not pressed to decide. You will also have to decide whether to only use pasteurized donor milk from a milk bank, or if you are going to engage in peer to peer sharing. Donor milk has risks, just like formula, and usually comes with a different set of emotional responses when you consider giving another person's milk to your baby. There are also financial considerations, if you cannot get donor milk covered by your insurance it is very expensive. Peer to peer milk is usually donated in exchange for pumping parts rather than purchased and this is to remove incentive to water it down or add volume by adding alternative milks in order to gain more profit. Some benefits of donor milk include involving partner in feeding, and baby getting a larger variety of antibodies and stem cells to strengthen his immune system and body, overall.

While using formula is not without risk, I believe the risks are misinterpreted or twisted sometimes to meet lactivist agendas. Studies show that infants who are not breastfed have higher rates of ear infections, stomach bugs, lung disease, obesity, diabetes, cancer, and SIDs. Premature infants who do not get breastmilk have an increased risk of bowel death. Females who do not breastfeed have higher rates of breast and ovarian cancer, obesity, diabetes, and metabolic syndrome (and thus the chronic illnesses that follow those diseases). This data does not say "formula fed babies," it says, "babies who do not get breastmilk," and "females who do not breastfeed." This leads me to interpret this as saying that any amount of breastmilk and any breastfeeding provide some protection against these things. The benefits of breastmilk are not proven to be dose-dependent, and there is no research on babies who are fed both formula and breastmilk. There is no data on females who breastfeed and formula feed simultaneously. It is my belief that any breastfeeding is providing all the protection and all the benefits to both the lactating parent and the baby, and we should be more flexible in allowing formula to help us meet the demands of infant feeding. When we pretend it is evil or not an option, we miss the gifts it is offering.

Not considering the need to supplement before delivery can make it feel like a much heavier decision when you are freshly postpartum and more sensitive than usual. In this case it is wise to hope for the best outcome but prepare for alternatives. It can negatively influence when you later reflect on the first few days of your baby's life if you feel pushed or rushed into the decision. Once you decide to supplement, or accept that you need to, you will also have to consider the tools you will use to supplement with.

Choices for supplementation include bottles, syringes, cups, at breast supplemental nursing systems (SNS), and finger feeding. When the need to supplement is in the first few days and in smaller quantities it can make sense to use anything but the bottles. Small syringes with curved tips are great for the first few days because you can have the baby suckle the breast or a finger while syringing some supplement into their cheeks. Finger feeding can be done with a syringe and tube set-up as well. Very small cups are also used worldwide to help pour small amounts into baby's mouth to get them to drink. This can be especially helpful if you have a baby with oral aversions who is resistant to latching onto anything.

Supplemental nursing systems (SNS) were invented to help adoptive mothers stimulate milk supply but can also be helpful for parents with low supply, premature infants, or babies who are full term but small for gestational age (SGA). They enable you to bring the baby to the breast while getting a supplement at the same time. They are made up of a bottle, bag, or syringe that connects to a tube. The reservoir holds the supplement and the tube tucks into the baby's mouth once they are suckling on the breast. This encourages the baby to keep suckling on the breast because they get a constant flow from the supplement.

Keep all of these options in mind if you need to supplement, as what you prefer may change over time. Once you are giving more than an ounce at a time to supplement, typically after the first few days, then some of these options can be cumbersome and not worth the minimal risk of nipple or flow preference that is present when you supplement temporarily with bottles. Many babies are happy to continue nursing even when they also need to supplement part time, which makes returning to the breast full time easier. The supplemental nursing system is often reserved for those we know will be supplementing for several months and prefer to keep baby at breast rather than use a bottle. Some parents find they prefer to use bottles because of the difficulty keeping the tubing in baby's mouth once they are more active. When bottle feeding it is important to use slow flow nipples and pace the feeding so that it mimics a breastfeeding session. It is of course possible to use a combination of supplementation techniques, depending on your preferences. In the first few weeks most babies are flexible on what supplemental device they will accept.

Many families find they prefer to keep some supplementation or bottle feeding once they have experienced the benefits of hybrid feeding. It allows more partner involvement, more rest for the breastfeeding parent, more flexibility for the whole family, and reduced stress around achieving and maintaining a full supply.

Gastrointestinal Disorders and Allergies

Most parents are concerned about reflux and food allergies. They are actually less common than most people believe. Many parents think that normal spit up patterns are signs of reflux, but in fact the two are very different. When it is reflux versus spit up, we often see a poor weight gain and the spit up is accompanied by signs of pain in the infant. Diagnosis of reflux must be done by a professional, and not an assumption by parents. Reflux and food allergies change the dynamics of breastfeeding and call for professional involvement. Food allergies might cause some physical symptoms in the baby like rashes, or poor weight gain.

Parents of infants with food allergies must remove the triggers from their diet, and sometimes it takes months of trial and error. Malabsorption, inborn metabolic errors, or inability to digest breastmilk are super rare and might mean you will have to formula feed, usually very special and expensive formulas. Some people might erroneously label these conditions as an allergy to breastmilk, but they are different than the process of an allergic response. An allergic response to breastmilk is usually due to an underlying food allergy and elimination of the food from the parent's diet can allow the breastfeeding relationship to continue. It is important that testing has confirmed whatever condition is suspected, and it is not just a suspicion. Many breastfeeding relationships could have been saved had testing been done, or an IBCLC involved in troubleshooting before jumping to specialized formulas. If you are facing being told to try special formulas and stop nursing, it is best to keep pumping to protect your supply so it is still available if it wasn't a breastmilk digestion problem, after all. In addition, your pumped and frozen breastmilk can be fed later if the child outgrows the allergy. Usually a trial of a few weeks on the special formula helps rule out some of these possibilities. You also likely have time to weed out triggering foods from your diet before switching to formula, as long as baby is stable and safe.

Anomalies

Any anatomical variations or changes to the nerves, nasal passages, face, cheeks, lips, neck, tongue, jaw, throat, heart, lungs, and gastrointestinal tract could be impactful to breast-feeding. The structure and the function must be normal in each place for the whole system of feeding to work. This includes a healthy heart and lungs because they have to keep up with the work of eating. There are so many body parts and systems involved in feeding, it would be beyond the scope of this book to review all of them in detail. The newborn is using multiple cranial nerves, bones, muscles, and reflexes to eat, and all of these are evaluated during a breastfeeding assessment.

Many babies with anomalies are erroneously categorized as lazy. Infants are not lazy; they cannot choose to be lazy. They act on instinct and if they are falling asleep quickly at the breast without getting enough to eat, it is because they are exerting a tremendous amount of energy trying to eat. If this sleepiness at the breast is excessive or interfering with weight gain, then the baby needs to be thoroughly assessed.

In the development of the oral cavity, babies can be born with oral anomalies like a large tongue, a small jaw, a cleft palate, cleft lip, and oral tethers. Anomalies that effect feeding can develop in otherwise healthy babies, but sometimes are linked to certain syndromes. These changes can make it difficult or impossible to create a seal, maintain a negative pressure suction, and simultaneously move the tongue thoroughly to remove the milk.

The structural anatomy and movements needed to move the mouth, tongue, and jaw are complex and varied during breastfeeding. Oral tethers are anomalies of connective tissue that prohibit full range of motion of the oral tissues, especially important are tethers found under the tongue and upper lip.

We all have connective tissue under our tongue, lips, and cheeks; sometimes that tissue is too tight, thick, or short, and it keeps the mouth and tongue from moving the way that they should. Tethers are treatable and you should work with a professional familiar with oral tethers if you suspect your baby has one. Some of the early signs of oral tethers are as follows: latch pain, shallow latch despite proper technique, "lipstick" nipple shape after nursing, damaged nipples, nipple damage that does not heal within the first week, reoccurring nipple infections, reoccurring clogs and mastitis, poor milk transfer, tiring easily at the breast, frustration at the breast, falling asleep quickly on the breast, reflux, excessive gas, choking on the letdown, excessively long feeds, unusually frequent feeds, lip blisters, low supply as a result of the poor milk transfer, not draining the breasts, and usually poor weight gain. An oral tether under the top lip, commonly called a lip tie, can keep the baby from opening their mouth wide enough, and prevent them from maintaining a seal with their lips. The lip will not flange out properly, and will tuck under itself because of the tension. Most babies with lip tie also have tongue tie, and the symptom lists are similar.

Additionally, your baby may start off breastfeeding decently and then suddenly do poorly around 3 months, this is often a sign of a missed diagnosis for oral tethers. Your supply regulation is largely hormonally driven the first 12 weeks postpartum so a person with a particularly good flow and abundant supply can compensate for what a baby's mouth cannot do for milk removal. When supply regulates more closely with what baby can remove from the breast around 3 months, if the mouth cannot do its job then the supply tanks and baby stops gaining weight well.

Often a restricted infant has a recessed jaw and narrow palate due to the fascia pulling the jaw back and preventing the tongue from making full contact with the roof of the mouth. Connection and suction between the tongue and the roof of the mouth allows for the cranial bones to develop with enough space for the teeth on the top jaw, without that connection there is a narrower palate than is needed. The bottom jaw is pulled back farther than it should be and the teeth are pulled inward as they grow in on the bottom jaw due to the tether repeatedly lifting the floor of the mouth with attempting full range of motion for speech and eating. These influences on anatomy lead to the adult teeth crowding, often requiring expensive dental and orthodontic work to try to correct the misalignments of the jaw and the crowding of the teeth. Headgear or surgery is often the treatment for the recessed jaw, which is much more expensive and painful than a frenotomy. While this might seem mostly cosmetic it is actually a matter of oral health, as crowded teeth lead to more cavities and an improper bite can lead to grinding and jaw pain.

Additionally, the range of motion of the tongue is restricted when the infant is learning to speak and eat. Tongue tied toddlers are often extremely picky eaters and will gag easily and choke on their food. Tongue tied toddlers also often need speech therapy. It is always better, when we have the option, to prevent an issue than to go back and try to fix it after the damage has occurred; in this scenario a frenotomy and the follow up care are less time consuming and expensive compared to years of speech therapy 1 to 3 times per week. There is no way of knowing if a tongue tie will affect speech, but the more anterior it is (towards the front of the tongue), the more likely it is to impact speech. With a posterior tie the front of the tongue still has a lot of range of motion to be able to make more sounds and speak more clearly.

Looking further into development ties can continue to impact quality of life and inhibit optimal development. As the facial structures grow tongue tied adults and children often find difficulty with proper breathing, especially when asleep. Common complaints and conditions of tongue-tied people are around snoring, not sleeping well, and having poor posture to try to breathe well. Children who do not sleep well often exhibit dysfunctional behaviors during the day like poor attention span, destructive tendencies, and crankiness. Tied babies and children often wake more frequently at night than is average.

Adolescents and adults with untreated tethers often have unhealthy gums, poor posture, frequent headaches, migraines, clicking or pain in the jaw, a locking jaw, sleep apnea, neck and back pain, and many other complaints. Most adults that seek revision, bodywork, and myotherapy wish they had done it earlier in life.

It is never too late in life to correct the tether with a revision, and in my opinion it is best to do as soon as the tether is diagnosed. An ounce of prevention is worth a pound of cure! There are more exhaustive lists available online of all the things that oral tethers can affect. The entirety of data around oral tethers would be outside of the scope of this book, but I wanted to highlight some of the most important possible effects.

You do always have the option not to revise a tether, but if it is affecting breastfeeding it will likely affect other things later in life. Breastfeeding is the first test of whether or not the tongue is functioning like it should. Another part of the information that is critical to this decision process is knowing what happens to untreated oral tethers, which is why I reviewed some of the possible outcomes. As development continues with a tether in place more compensation for the restriction develops, more bodily functions are affected, and the development of the anatomy is influenced. Weight gain being the deciding factor for revision is very short-sighted and is sadly often what providers and parents base their decision on; that is why I found it so important to expand past beyond how it affects breastfeeding in this book.

If your baby has an oral tether you do have other options outside of just revising or not revising. If you want to watch and wait rather than rush to treat, it is never too late to treat a tether. There are rare cases where babies cannot even gain weight well on bottles because of oral tethers, and typically in those cases the benefits to revision more clearly present themselves as greater than the risks. So, unless it is life threatening, revising a tether is usually at parental discretion. Your child will not outgrow it, but the body will learn to compensate. Usually, this compensation comes at a cost such as tension and pain, as well as all of the symptoms of tongue tie; some which present right away and some that present later in life. Sometimes with breastfeeding, small adjustments can be made such as using a nipple shield, which allows for some compensation as it helps hold the nipple in the mouth; this however is only a band-aid and is a temporary solution to a chronic problem.

Then there is also the consideration of method of revision. Some parents might find, after they decide to pursue a frenotomy or frenectomy, they need to choose between a provider that uses a laser and a provider that uses scissors. Most tongue tie savvy professionals will agree, what matters more is experience and skill. The provider who releases the tie should be knowledgeable, thorough, experienced, aware of possible risks and benefits to both doing the procedure and not, aware of posterior restriction (not just anterior), promote body work in conjunction with revision, and promote proper wound care protocols, such as stretching the wound post-revision.

Feelings and responses to the suggestion of revision are varied. Sometimes parents know right away they want to do it. Sometimes they want time to think about it. Sometimes parents would rather pump or formula feed. You may find your partner comes to a different conclusion about the necessity of revision than you, and that might cause tension or stress. The responses to tethers from parents and the options available are just as varied as the responses you might get from various professionals.

I believe what is most important is that you are making an educated decision and that your healthcare providers respect you. In most cases though, there is time to decide. Use that time to educate yourself and weigh long term risks versus benefits.

I would not be doing my job if I did not inform you here of the fact that oral tethers are a heavily debated topic amongst professionals, and treatment has become a political pawn in many communities. Reviewing some of the history around its diagnosis and treatment will help shed light on why. There is historical evidence that we have treated tongue ties for at least five-hundred years. We treated it long enough and often enough that now a large portion of the population has it, as it is typically genetically carried. In recent history, oral tethers such as obvious anterior (front of the mouth) tongue ties were clipped by midwives immediately after delivery. When obstetricians took over birth, they stopped this practice because they deemed it barbaric, likely because most midwives did it using their pinky nail. Obviously, presently sterile tools are used, and consent is obtained. This timing of birth practice changes was a perfect storm with formula being heavily marketed and pushed as superior to breast milk. These changes lining up eventually led to oral tethers not commonly being treated in newborns and being left out of medical school curriculum; because there was no breastfeeding problem that formula could not fix! It essentially went out of style to fix them in infants for the past 80-100 years, yet they continued to be passed on genetically. Many will say treating tethers is a fad, but in fact the opposite is true. The fad was not treating them and favoring formula. As we swing back the other direction and find a happy middle ground, there will be turbulence in the medical community. Most currently practicing professionals while well-meaning and well-educated do not know how to adequately assess for or treat tongue ties, nor understand their potential chronic impacts. This is through no fault of their own, just lack of consensus and adequate training availability. Many who are oral tether knowledgeable have gone above and beyond their basic education to learn more about them.

Oral tethers like lip and tongue ties are definitely an area where you will get conflicting professional opinions. The resurgence of concern over oral tethers has ruffled a lot of physician's feathers—because they do not get trained adequately in medical school about their impact and when treatment is needed. They most especially do not understand how they impact breastfeeding. Even some lactation consultants will deny they are a problem. When you come across a large group of pediatricians who are not trained on ties and they have a large stake in a local hospital's business they might put a gag-order of sorts on the nurses, having administration threaten to fire them if they suggest to parents that their baby might have them. What this means for parents is that you will get various professionals with various training giving you various opinions. It can make being the parent of a tethered baby very frustrating and confusing.

As medicine has advanced in the past few decades, oral tethers have been found to need to be released by other specialties. Other professionals started releasing oral tethers in toddlers, children, adolescents, and adults for dentition, orthodontics, speech and language pathology, feeding difficulties, headaches, sleep disturbances, breathing difficulties, migraines, lockjaw, and other issues. In recent decades, these specialists began wondering: why did we stop preventing these problems by releasing these ties in infants? There is no doubt with an understanding of human anatomy and development that an oral tether influences many systems. Many adult tongue tie patients often express they wish their parents had corrected their tether in infancy or childhood, and are not discovering their tethers until their own children or grandchildren are diagnosed.

There is still argument and lack of data on how prevalent oral tethers are, how often they might need treatment, and if preventative treatment is advisable for the potential issues later in life. The modern assessment and treatment of oral tethers is still a developing science. There is a lack of quality published research demonstrating evidence of the questions that parents want answered. Much of the lack of data is due to the lack of studies being done. There is not solid contrary evidence to these anatomical development theories, nor is there evidence showing a lack of benefits of treatment.

Risks of revision are often similar to any procedure. The procedure might not produce the desired results, the procedure might need repeated, the procedure might cause excessive bleeding, and there is risk of infection. Typically, bleeding is minimal to none, and infection is exceedingly rare as the mouth is so quick to heal, and breastmilk has antibodies to kill bacteria. An exhaustive list of potential risks and benefits would have to be personalized for each baby. It would be based on the baby's medical history, the provider, the technique, and the suggested aftercare.

Revision of a tongue tie does not and cannot guarantee breastfeeding success, and for most babies takes many weeks of retraining their tongue to eventually nurse efficiently. Expecting it to be a quick fix because it is a quick and low risk procedure will set you up for disappointment. Additionally, it is important to note that some babies are also not good candidates for revision, for example when they have poor muscle tone.

A tongue tie revision should be accompanied by suck training and body work to support all of the muscles involved in feeding, because the baby has been practicing suckling with restriction in utero for many weeks. Body work includes chiropractic, craniosacral therapy, physical therapy, occupational therapy, speech therapy, orofacial myology, and massage. Your baby might not need help from all of these specialists but will likely need at least 1-3 supporting therapies to improve the function of the tongue. Optimal functioning after revision is often realized 4 to 6 weeks after the procedure. Sometimes things get worse during healing, as the body attempts to reconnect the severed tissues. This is especially true when the baby's muscles are most sore post procedure day 3 to 5, and then again with healing tension around day 7 to 10. This is why your baby should be on a wound stretching protocol. Usually, this means doing a few steps before feeds, like swiping under the tongue, and pushing up the tongue with two fingers towards the roof of the mouth. There are great resources online detailing post-frenotomy care, so I will not say much more about it here. Your provider should be the one to offer a detailed plan for your child, these are just possible examples. Staying on top of stretches, exercises, massage, and other body work will help you get past the phases where the healing tissue attempts to reattach or tighten up again. Things might get worse rather than better if you do not have a comprehensive and team approach after frenotomy; just clipping the tie alone will not fix all of the issues. Part of your team should be an IBCLC, to assess improvements in milk transfer and latch pain, as you might need to adjust your typical positioning and latch methods, or need to pursue a second revision if the first was not deep enough, or it reattaches.

Tongue tie is on a spectrum of severity, but they are present, or not. A tongue tie is not mild just because an infant can compensate using a nipple shield. The behavior of the tongue and the quality of the breastfeeding relationship without extraneous tools is the true picture of function. If a tongue-tied baby is requiring an elaborate and laborious feeding process in order to gain weight, then the tie is a problem. If a baby has unexplained colic or reflux, those might be symptoms of a tie. And no, babies do not grow out of them, and they do not stretch out. They type of collagen that the frenulum is made of never stretches out, it will be the tissue and bone around the restriction that give-way, and that is usually at a cost.

Some of the providers you discuss tongue tie with will get heated or make it personal or try to scare you (from both sides of the isle). It is safest to seek multiple opinions, and from multiple specialties, and ask the professionals to explain to you in detail their assessment of the oral cavity. Simply looking in the mouth or glancing under the tongue is not a proper assessment. Assessing how far the tongue can stick out is a common assessment, and it is woefully inadequate as it only shows a single range of motion. The tongue needs to cup to seal the areola in place with the help of the lips, and then also undulate to draw out the milk. All of which only has partially to do with extension. If they are not assessing multiple motions of the tongue, they are not providing a thorough assessment. Providers should also be able to explain in detail why a procedure called revision or frenectomy is recommended, or not. I have linked in my "resources" section how to find what are called "preferred providers" that will have had extra training above and beyond what was required in school to learn more about oral tethers, and have good reputations as being trustworthy and competent when treatment is needed. There is also information and feedback available from other parents of their experiences with these providers.

Baby's issues with feeding

Commonly a baby with difficulty getting milk flow at the breast will develop a preference for bottles. This is often mistakenly called nipple confusion. Babies are not confused—they want the milk the easiest and most comfortable way they can get it. I believe they develop a flow preference. When they have an easier time getting a flow and getting full from the bottle, they will prefer it. Preferring the easiest way to get food is likely a survival instinct. Using a slow flowing nipple bottle and paced feeding techniques can somewhat help a baby to not prefer the bottle over the breast.

A baby that can latch comfortably and can stimulate fast gushes of milk via the let-down is going to be happy at the breast. A baby will also be happy at the breast if milk flow is abundant even without much effort on their part to draw the milk out. If a baby is either sleeping at the breast after a short period of suckling or angry at the breast, then they are signaling that there is a problem with flow, and many parents think they do this because they are waiting for or demanding a bottle. These issues could be because baby cannot efficiently remove the milk, or it may be because the milk flow is too slow or low to keep him happy and interested, or it could be both.

Many parents also mistake normal milk stimulating actions as refusal of the breast, and rush too quickly to give the bottle. All mammals pop on and off the nipple, shake their head, and fuss and "paw" at the breast or teat. It looks like the baby is pushing the breast away, but they are trying to knead it. Shaking their head is not saying "no" it is how they help stimulate the nipple to erect position. This is all on purpose and helps stimulate the letdown. As long as baby is not angry it is important to let them exhibit this natural and instinctive behavior on the breast. Watch videos of baby led latching, as well as puppies and kitties nursing, to get an idea of what I mean.

Bottle preference developing when the nursing parent is at work for many hours a week is usually due to the caretaker making the bottle too fast, too large, and too often. The parent cannot keep up with the overfeeding because it is outside of the biological norm, and baby becomes accustomed to the new changes and prefers them because they are getting full faster and easier. The pace, frequency, and volume being too much are not because the parent is failing to pump enough but because the caretaker is doing little to soothe the baby other than offering a bottle. Discussing "paced" feeding techniques and appropriate amounts with your infant's caregiver should take place as early as possible to help manage expectations to avoid unintentional sabotage of the breastfeeding relationship. This is an important discussion to have, sometimes repeatedly, with whomever will be feeding your baby when you are at work. They will need to know what resources they have, tools they can use, and skills they need to develop to soothe a fussy baby, other than just giving them a bottle.

Pumping

Some babies cannot or will not latch and breastfeed due to a myriad of other reasons, sometimes an undiagnosed or missed issue. Some develop oral aversion and are hard to feed, even with a bottle. Some are simply too impatient or frustrated at the breast due to sensory processing disorders. You want the breast to be a happy and stress-free space and to minimize putting anything in the baby's mouth aside from a flowing breast. Minimize does not mean avoid entirely, so please do not confuse this with advice like "avoid a bottle at all costs!" I have seen many babies take the breast and the bottle easily, it just has to be handled strategically. Early challenges with babies that will not latch or cannot latch might necessitate exclusive pumping or minimal breastfeeding if you desire to continue to provide breast milk. These babies are good candidates for a feeding specialist referral. If your baby does develop a bottle preference, or resistance to the breast, you can work with a lactation consultant and feeding specialist to coax them back to the breast.

I have seen many parents successfully bring a non-latching preemie or baby to the breast after several months of pumping. What works for the first few days, few weeks, or few months might change as your baby grows. Often, when a bottle-fed baby switches to at the breast feeding, they are a bit older. It is common for them to lean out, too, as they are better able to self-regulate their intake at the breast versus when bottle fed. This is true even though the substance in the bottle is breastmilk. If you find yourself pumping and bottle feeding but still wanting to feed from the breast, check in with your IBCLC once a month to assess baby's latch and milk transfer, and get tips to bring baby to the breast.

Nursing aversions are one reason that might necessitate exclusive pumping or minimal feeding at the breast. Sometimes the aversion is temporary, and we would call it a nursing strike. Conversely, it is also possible that your baby might refuse bottles or go on bottle strikes. Severe oral aversions or anomalies may lead to your baby needing nasal-gastric tube feeding or a more permanent tube inserted directly into the stomach. Some of the root causes of oral aversion are sensory processing disorder, trauma, or oral anomalies.

Exclusive pumping to provide breast milk is an option for some parents when direct latching does not work out, or a parent is uncomfortable with direct latching. It can be one way to meet your goals of breastfeeding. Pumping is still breastfeeding, as you are feeding milk from the breast. However, it is important to note that some people do not respond well to pumps and are unable to make this option work.

Exclusive pumping as an option for feeding for most parents means around the clock hooking up to a machine and being tied to a wall for 15-20 minutes every 2-3 hours for the first 2-3 months while supply regulates. Later on, around 4-6 months you might be able to reduce the pump sessions to every 3-4 hours and maintain the same daily output.

If you are fortunate you might be able to get the new style of pumps that allow you to walk around and get things done while you pump. Several versions are out now that are covered by insurance. There are even breast shaped flanges that can sit in the bra, making it difficult to see that you are even pumping—aside from the connecting tubes to the small pump. These portable pumps have traditional flanges, but the pump motor is on a necklace or hip clip. Several of the more expensive pumps do not even have any cords or strings and the entire system simply pops into the bra. This is a modernization of pumps that is long overdue and really should be available to everyone, but for now is a luxury and only covered by some insurances and not always at 100%. Choosing which pump to get can feel overwhelming, so this might be something you discuss with a consultant or start investigating while you are pregnant.

Exclusive pumping can be harder than nursing in many ways. It often follows a few days or weeks of frustration and exhaustion from trying to get nursing to work. It is harder to respond to a pump hormonally and emotionally in the same way you do to a latched baby and is thus harder to maintain supply. It can also be hard because it can tempt you to obsess over numbers. It also feels quite different emotionally to do a mechanical task with a machine versus a bonding, interactive, and connected moment with an infant. Your pump membranes and valves will need replaced more frequently than if you were only pumping some of the time, which can add expenses. Additionally, even if you are committed and enthusiastic about pumping it is hard to maintain that resolve. It is also unlikely to be successful if you do not start out exclusively pumping and then attempt to switch to it several months later, as it is harder to respond to a pump the further postpartum you are --especially if you did not train your breasts to respond to pumps when your supply was largely hormonally driven in the first 12 weeks.

Some practical things that can help with pumping include using as many of your senses as possible to encourage a stronger hormonal response. Simulating as many things as you can about feeding at the breast will help do this. To imitate a warm and wriggling baby, place warmers on your chest and massage your breasts; this engages your sense of temperature and sense of touch. The massaging is similar to how babies knead the breast to help encourage flow. If you cannot get a pumping bra to help make this step easier, try making one by cutting holes in an old bra, tank top, or tube top. To engage your sight and hearing, watch videos of your baby; if they are crying, even better. Crying tends to trigger a let-down. To mimic the baby's mouth, you should warm and lubricate the pump flange, because your body will respond better to this than cold hard plastic. Finally, engage your sense of smell. Smelling your baby, or their hats and blankets, while you pump activates a strong hormonal response that encourages your body to make milk. You can even include your sense of taste by being sure to eat and drink when pumping, as some studies have shown that doing so boosts production.

Of course, with exclusive pumping usually comes exclusive bottle feeding, which harbors its own set of challenges. Staying on top of cleaning the parts, finding the right bottle, facing judgement, self-deprecating thoughts, and negative emotions around bottle feeding are just some of the potential challenges. Some parents find they resent the labor around pumping and bottle-feeding when they are grieving, because they would rather be directly nursing. Alternatively, of course, many find the freedom and predictability of bottle feeding to be preferential to feeding at the breast.

Sometimes babies need to be fed by tubes. Tube feeding might look like a tube that goes down through the nose and into the stomach, or a tube that is surgically placed on the abdomen, with a cap that closes and opens for access. When this is the case, parents have to learn complicated and technical medical techniques and procedures to ensure this is done safely and correctly. The NICU team will usually teach you what you need to know before you are discharged from the hospital, your insurance will provide supplies and possibly a home health nurse to help, and you will have close and frequent follow up with your feeding specialists team. Some babies that start out tube feeding end up going on the breast or bottle feed, and the opposite can be true, too. Missed diagnoses, late presenting genetic conditions, failure to thrive, accidents, oral aversions, and other events might lead to your team deciding tube fed is best until your baby can thrive with oral feedings.

Many parents who end up exclusive pumping feel they had little choice, but still wanted to provide milk for their baby. Without proper support and sometimes missed diagnoses, parents are pushed or forced into thinking pumping is the only option when all options have not actually been explored. This might leave you with the task of grieving what you wanted and making peace with what is. If you have a suspicion more could be done or assessed, do not be afraid to advocate for your breastfeeding relationship. You may need to ask for a referral to an infant feeding specialist or go see multiple professionals to get second, third, or fourth opinions! It is also okay if you do not have the emotional energy to keep pushing for it to work, and ultimately decide not to nurse. Most people cannot imagine how hard and heavy that feels until faced with it. I think knowing this is a potential reality ahead of time can help soften the blow.

You may choose from the beginning to exclusively pump, so the emotional challenge of the choice might not apply to you. It is important that you know it is logistically and hormonally harder to maintain your supply. It can also be harder to continue to resolve to meet your goal when you are sick of being stuck to a wall for 15 minutes every 2-3 hours for an entire year. Those times can sometimes feel like you are missing out on things and are stretched too thin with all your other responsibilities. It is also rare to respond to a pump after 1 year postpartum, so do not count on exclusive pumping for a goal of over 1 year of providing milk. There is also the risk of the frozen stored milk being ruined by a freezer breaking, a natural disaster, or an absent-minded family member leaving the freezer door ajar. Additionally, it can be harder to have to carry around and manage all the equipment for pumping and bottle feeding. Even with the differences, some find exclusive pumping more convenient.

Pumping, exclusively or partially, is often part of the modern breastfeeding relationship. For many parents it is initially a stressor and is being used because something with breastfeeding is not going well. You might fret over how little comes out at first. It is more about the stimulation than the amount. You will have to trouble shoot, and figure things out with trial and error. It can also be stressful to learn how to use a new machine when you are more exhausted than you have ever been in your life. You will also need to learn about proper milk storage. This might be something you want to know about before the baby comes.

While proper milk storage guidelines are available many places online, I will summarize them here. Freshly expressed breastmilk is good at room temperature for 4 to 6 hours. After that, milk should be moved to the fridge, and then kept any-where from 3 to 7 days depending on its smell and taste. If you are not going to use that milk, then you can freeze it. In a regularly used freezer the milk is good for 3 months in a door, and 6 months if kept deeper in the back or bottom. In a deep freezer that is opened less often, you can keep it for 12 months. Studies of frozen milk do not suggest that it spoils while frozen, but some of the nutrients start to be broken down, making the milk slightly less nutritious. Once milk has touched the baby's mouth it is only good another few hours, so maybe until the next feeding if they are close together. This is different from formula, which has to be tossed within an hour. Once frozen milk is thawed, it should be used within 24 hours. Once heated, it is not recommended to heat and cool breastmilk multiple times because it encourages bacterial growth. Some families feel comfortable going outside of these suggestions if the milk still smells and tastes good, and if you do so it is at your own risk. The guidelines are meant to help keep the bacterial count in the milk down, to avoid spoiling or food poisoning. Since breastmilk is living with antibodies, it can kill bacteria and slow the growth of it, so that makes this a tricky science.

Often when things are not going well initially most con-sultants will put you on a breast, bottle, pump plan. Sometimes this is called triple-feeding. This is doing all 3 things at every feed, every 2-3 hours, around the clock. This is ridiculously hard logistically and can go on for weeks—especially with a preemie. Be prepared to do some hard work up front so that you can get to the smooth sailing later on, that is exclusive breastfeeding. Most parents only have to do the triple feeding plan for less than a week. Premature infants are often ready to transition when they are at their due date, or about 4 weeks after. You should be having close follow ups to get off the plan, or reduce the plan, as soon as possible.

In the early postpartum weeks is also typically when parents pursue circumcisions, if that is something they have decided to do or if it needs done for medical reasons. Babies will typically sleep prolonged amounts of time compared to normal when they are recovering. This might necessitate some extra pumping and bottle feeding temporarily. Some parents find circumcision interrupts the establishment of the nursing relationship.

When you are breastfeeding full time or part time, you might be hit with a nursing strike. Nursing strikes that are temporary typically develop later on in the relationship, rather than in the early days. A nursing strike might necessitate exclusive pumping for a few days, while waiting for baby to come back to the breast. Sometimes the strike is only for one breast, but not both. Breastfeeding can be going well, and something might startle the baby on the breast or change the way breastfeeding is feeling. Examples might be a strong maternal reaction to being bitten, or an ear infection causing pain while laying on one side. It would be important to protect your supply by replacing that stimulation with pumping and keep offering the breast with gentle and low-stress strategies. Be prepared for the rejection to hurt your feelings.

These are usually temporary and can be worked through. This is often mistaken for "early weaning" but babies will rarely truly wean from the breast before 1 year of age. Toddlers can even be brought back to the breast, for example, after strikes through subsequent pregnancies. This is because they do not appreciate the flavor change or the decreased volumes during pregnancy but are often happy to resume at the breast when the baby comes, and the milk is flowing again. Pumping through a nursing strike while pregnant would not preserve supply, because the placenta would be hormonally controlling the supply and causing the breasts to only make colostrum.

Baby Behaviors That Can be Challenging

There are certain behaviors at the breast that are developmentally appropriate but cringe-worthy, annoying, and frustrating. Babies might be distracted during feeds, violent at the breast, twiddle your nipples, or bite you.

Nursing violence is just another issue parents face. It is when your baby inflicts violence upon your person while they are nursing. Of course, they are not trying to hurt you—but they do. They are often exploring what their bodies can do or trying to elicit letdowns. Just go ahead and put away that picture in your mind of beautiful Madonna and child nursing peacefully.

Babies often scratch you and pinch you. They are born with talons. Their instinctive behavior as newborns is much like a puppy or kitty that you will see pawing at the teat. Babies work the breast by pinching and kneading in order to help the milk flow. The kneading can present like they are pushing you away, which sometimes can hurt your feelings if you do not understand what they are trying to do. Many parents struggle with allowing the baby to follow these instincts. Many prefer wrapping them up in a swaddle to avoid the wrestling match, or to cover their sharp nails with mittens.

When your flow is strong or the latch is shallow, they might choke or gag, which is scary and unsettling. When they get older, they may kick you and slap you, and just generally wriggle around while they eat. As they get more curious, they stick their fingers in your nose and mouth to check things out. When they are in a distractible developmental phase, they may pull your nipple sideways as they try to look away—yet stay latched. Although maybe not violent, older infants and toddlers also engage in gym-nurstics, which is when they contort their body into various poses while nursing. Not to mention, it is not violence but highly frustrating, in the distractible phase when they unlatch frequently to look around. Nursing in a nice quiet and dark space for most feeds helps diminish this, but that can be logistically challenging to do at every single feeding, especially when you have other children.

Twiddling is its own special brand of nursing violence that many parents endure. Pinching and pulling your other nipple while nursing on the opposite side helps stimulate letdowns for babies. This can be especially tough if you have sensitive nipples or just do not particularly like your nipples tweaked. Twiddling is an extremely hard habit to break, so try to avoid developing it to begin with by keeping only one breast exposed at a time. This may not entirely curb the behavior, as they may still try to stick their hand down your shirt. Some will refuse to keep nursing unless they are allowed to engage in twiddling.

Teething itself is not violent but can lead to some biting, which is. Babies often bite for teething comfort, but sometimes they bite for other reasons. They might bite down as a last-ditch effort to stimulate a milk flow if their tongue is not doing the trick. They might bite down if the flow is too strong and they are trying to block it. They might bite down just to see how you will react.

Teething can also change the saliva and lead to more frequent comfort nursing which will cause some sore nipples, even without biting. A proper and deep latch will prevent a baby from being able to bite down. If the latch is deep the gums will be over the areola which is less sensitive than the nipple. Additionally, the tongue should be covering the lower gumline making it difficult to feel an impact on the lower side of the bite. The best thing to do is watch your baby carefully for signs they might be about to bite and break the latch before they do. Biting phases are usually truly short.

Another baby behavior that can be challenging is when they do not take to solids well. If you were anticipating weaning by a certain age but your baby is not eating solids well enough then you might continue to nurse. Often while working through this many parents are told to wean to make the child hungrier, but this can backfire. If it is an issue that is causing the need for therapists to help encourage your child to eat, then taking away the milk will give them even less opportunity to get the nutrition they need. There is often a push and pull with this dynamic of being glad you can provide the sustenance with a frustration around your baby not moving on from breastfeeding as quickly or as progressively as you had hoped. When this gets into two to three years of age, many parents find themselves feeling tapped-out or resentful. If you feel like your baby is not eating like they should, seek help from your healthcare village. Difficulty with eating solids can be discussed with the occupational therapist, speech therapist, tongue tie specialist, and chiropractor. Keep pushing for progress and answers if you need to.

Special Circumstances

Other special circumstances outside of the more typical lactating parent-infant dyad can add even more challenges. You might be facing breastfeeding multiple babies, decide to breast-feed a baby you did not give birth to, have a physical disability that makes the logistics of feeding challenging, be a teen parent, have multiple parents caring for one infant, have a premature infant, have an infant with health conditions that effect feeding, or not identify as a woman but decide to carry and nurse an infant if you're biologically able.

Breastfeeding multiple babies does not always mean you will face more troubles, but you will have twice the opportunity for challenges than a typical one to one parent-infant dyad. It is also often harder to build up enough supply for two babies, but not impossible. Multiples are also more likely to deliver prematurely than singletons. The good news is you do not have to do it without support!

Support is also needed if you are a parent that needs to induce lactation for a baby that you did not give birth to. Many people do not know this is possible, but any mammal with mammary tissue can make milk! Examples of when this might be beneficial include when two parents want to nurse their baby, or an adoptive parent wants to nurse her baby. There is sometimes stigma around nursing when a parent wishes to feed at the breast that is not the biological female or the parent who carried the child. There is an extensive protocol to follow for these cases and that takes several months, so you would definitely want professional guidance to optimize your plan.

Parents who have disabilites can face specific logistical challenges that other parents do not face. This will require creative problem solving and team work, but most lactating persons are able to provide milk if they want to. No chronic condition should be an automatic dismissal of attempting to breast-feed, if that is what the parent desires. Specifics would best be left to getting a thorough assessment from your healthcare team, especially your IBCLC, and then making a plan based on the level of support needed.

Teen parents also face more challenges than most parents due to the social stigma, logistical demands around returning to school, and financial concerns around supporting themselves and their baby if they have lost their family support. While many people assume teen parents will not breastfeed, many want to and most are successful when they have an adequate support system. Many teens have a harder time de-sexualizing the breasts, and getting comfortable with nursing. Once education and support are in place, there is a good chance that breast-feeding will go well. Most of the issues teen parents face outside of that are the same issues that other parents face. If financial or economic factors are a hinderance, there are many social programs and "mother's" homes that will help teen parents get off to a good start. The key is connecting with the right people to get resources, such as care coordinators, patient advocates, and care management nurses through the insurance, hospital, and government programs.

Some families have more than two parents, and this might be a time for growth and tension, as change often brings. You will want to talk about who is expected or willing to care for the infant, and re-define your roles within your relationship in relation to parenting your new baby. You might want to discuss if more than one parent will be nursing the infant, or if everyone is most comfortable with only one parent taking on that duty.

There is also the possibility that you prefer to refer to breast-feeding as chest-feeding. This can be frustrating to navigate when so many professionals in lactation are not in the habit of using that term. I can assure you there are plenty of lactation consultants who would be happy to support you if this is your circumstance, and would make the effort to support you in the way that you needed. It is often out of habit and deference that we automatically call feeding from the chest, "breastfeeding" and never intend to offend by calling it so. This is not meant to be exclusive or insensitive, it is the biological term and makes for easier readability and translation for non-native English speakers. When I refer to the breast it is because I mean the mound of fat and mammary tissue on the chest, and there is not another good name for that body part that most people recognize that is easily translatable. You might notice, I do use the word mamma (pronounced like the word mammary; mam-uh) or mammae (mam-ay) to describe the breast or breasts interchangeably to help bring that word back into circulation. It is currently obsolete in the English language, but might be a suitable substitute for those who prefer not to use "breast".

The term breastfeeding here is meant to be a catchall for lactating or feeding human milk, regardless of method of delivery. We require breast tissue to make breast milk, and breastfeeding includes any mode of feeding that milk. Feel free to think of the term chest feeding interchangeably anytime I refer to feeding from the breast if it makes you most comfortable. Breastfeeding is also interchangeable with pumping, because the milk is still coming from the breast. Additionally, I am aware not all people capable of carrying, birthing, and making milk for a child identify as a "woman," and I am actively working on practicing using more inclusive language such as using the word "parent" or "person," as well as using the word "female" when I am describing things unique to a genetically female body. In the same vein, I realize not all parents are only two people, and not all partners are male and female, and not all are married, so I try to refer to significant others as "partners." Please be patient with me on developing my inclusive language, I am trying.

The special circumstances around feeding a premature infant or one with health challenges as mentioned before creates more obstacles to overcome. It can be helpful to frame your mind around that getting to your goal might take longer, but it is generally possible for most dyads with persistence and professional guidance. Every baby deserves the chance to try. If you are told "most babies with this condition do not breastfeed" then it is time to ask for a personalized assessment of what your child is capable of. Do not let providers write off your child as unable to breastfeed unless they have done a thorough and comprehensive assessment of their ability to feed at the breast. More information around health concerns not covered in this chapter can be discussed with your specialist providers and an IBCLC who has a better understanding of your baby's health and diagnosis.

The Breastfeeding Relationship

Here we should cover most things about the breastfeeding relationship that you will need to consider while you are breast-feeding. Parents often want to know about food and drug safety while breastfeeding, getting sleep with a newborn, how breast-feeding works with also eating solids, nursing through physical and mental illness, what a normal breastfeeding relationship looks like, and how long they should aim to provide breastmilk for. We will explore each of these in depth.

Food Safety

One of the top concerns of parents is wondering if a specific food or drug is safe while breastfeeding. The good news is the rules about food while breastfeeding are much easier to follow than the rules about food during pregnancy. Many suggestions circulating about avoiding certain foods while breastfeeding are just myths. You really just want to avoid large amounts of alcohol, and a few specific herbs, because they can decrease supply. The herbs are fine in small doses for most people, such as flavoring for dishes, but individual responses vary. Herbs that can decrease supply should be avoided in oil or tea forms, or large quantities. Otherwise, eat normally. Yes, even spicy foods. The herbs that might decrease supply are jasmine, parsley, sage, peppermint, spearmint, menthol, lemon balm, oregano, thyme, black walnut, chickweed, and yarrow.

If your baby has rare food allergies that make it necessary for you to avoid certain foods then that will be diagnosed by a professional, and they will likely have several obvious symptoms like hives, blood in the stool, swelling, or red irritation around the mouth or anus. Fussiness, gassiness, frequent feeding, and pooping often are not symptoms of food allergies, just normal newborn behavior that is often erroneously attributed to food intolerances. Work with a professional if you are concerned. Though, even food allergists are not always lactation medicine savvy so take their lactation advice with a grain of salt. They will be able to diagnose what foods your child should avoid or tell you what is safe to have small dose exposure to. If they are suggesting the child is allergic, then you would cut it out of your diet for at least 4-6 weeks before re-introducing the foods one at a time to check for reactions.

The most common allergen or food sensitivity for babies is dairy. This often causes inflammation in adults, and we have consumed it for so many years that our symptoms go unnoticed. Biologically we are not designed as mammals to need milk after our milk teeth fall out, you might know them as baby teeth. In an infant when the cow dairy proteins irritate the stomach and intestines you will often see blood and mucous in the stool. Cutting dairy can be awfully hard, if needed. Not only is it a hidden ingredient in many foods but it is designed to be addictive, so that babies will continue to return for more and thus be more likely to survive. Many regions in our brain that light up with drugs also light up when we consume dairy products. Usually adults do just fine processing the bit of irritation dairy can cause, but babies might have a harder time. Other than the gastrointestinal upset, they might also struggle to gain weight or have signs on their skin like eczema. Be prepared that you might have to say goodbye to milkshakes and cheese for a while. The good news is that most babies outgrow the sensitivity in a few months.

Some professionals will suggest switching to formula for dairy intolerance, which blows my mind as formula is literally a dairy product. Switching to cow milk that is commercially altered into formula is not going to help symptoms of dairy intolerance. If that suggestion is made to you, you can safely assume you need to seek a second opinion.

The foods we eat do not usually dramatically alter the composition of our milk, as the body will draw from fat and mineral stores in your skin and bones if the diet is inadequate. You can influence the fat profile by having a variety of healthy fats, but not the quantity of fat. Good fats are found in salmon, sardines, eggs, olive oil, coconut oil, avocado, and nuts. Other important nutrients that we are typically low in are vitamin D and choline. Because we do not store these well, we need ongoing dietary sources. Good choline sources are eggs, liver, peanuts, meat, poultry, fish, dairy, or choline supplements. Good Vitamin D sources are fish and mushrooms, as well as some fortified foods, and of course supplements. The best supplements are all natural, and food sourced, or food based.

Most lactating people will do well to just have a varied, colorful, whole food diet. You do not need more than a few hundred extra calories, and maybe not even that if you have extra stored fat. High protein foods will help curb intense hunger and cravings. High protein can be meat, eggs, and nuts. Eating many colorful whole foods will help you get a variety of minerals and vitamins. It is important that you not dramatically change your diet or drastically reduce your calories while nursing, even when it seems that it is a healthier change. Changes should be slow, calculated, and gradual. Any shock to the system may result in a drop in supply.

It is also usually safe to follow cultural breastfeeding diet suggestions. While we have no evidence that they work, we also do not have any evidence saying they do not work or that they are unsafe. In general, these diets encourage adequate nutrition and hydration, and sometimes include foods that have some galactagogue qualities.

I believe another topic that falls under food safety is a discussion around hydration. Some people encourage lactating females to drink water in quite excessive amounts, insisting it helps increase supply. While it might temporarily improve the volume of the milk, it is just adding water not more nutritional content. Several studies have shown that drinking to thirst is adequate. So, if you are thirsty, drink. If you are not, do not make yourself. Avoiding drinks that dehydrate you like coffee and other caffeinated beverages helps. Drinking low sugar electrolyte drinks helps, too, because the electrolytes encourage your body to hold on to more water. There are no special, magical drinks that provide meaningful boosts in supply. Save those for when you are dehydrated from a stomach bug, or on your period.

You have to keep some tools in your back pocket for when you have inevitable supply dips, and not try to use them all every day for the whole first year of nursing. This is usually too expensive for most people, and it makes breastfeeding more stressful and challenging than it needs to be.

Drugs

Medications can be tricky because if you ask: "Is this safe for breastfeeding?" there is a different and separate answer for "Will this affect my supply?" Providers who do not work with breastfeeding dyads routinely will usually just tell you to "pump and dump" to be safe and so they might avoid liability. It is always up to you to investigate the safety and then the possible effect on supply. Many medications can affect your supply, and a good general understanding is that anything that dries things out, can dry up your milk. That includes decongestants and allergy medications. You should avoid aspirin, anything radio-active, anti-cancer, statins, immunosuppressive, and certain blood pressure medications; the list of what is dangerous is shorter than the list of what is safe, and there are almost always alternatives so be sure to always look it up and use all of your resources.

InfantRisk run by Dr. Thomas Hale at Texas Tech University (under "Resources" in this book) is the world class expert on drugs affecting pregnancy and breastfeeding. They have a website and hotline which are free, as well as a book and app for purchase.

It is a good sign if the professional you seek help from consults this or another trusted resource. Be wary of any feeding advice from a provider whom off-handedly suggests you pump-and-dump without actually looking up the information, and no, the manufacturer insert doesn't count. Cross check their suggestion with InfantRisk and do the next breastfeeding person they treat a favor and share that information with them. Sometimes providers knowledge is limited, and frankly they do not care about your breastfeeding relationship with the weight that you do, so it is wise to be skeptical. Very few drugs require weaning or interrupting breastfeeding.

Caffeine is the most used drug and is a hot topic, and many people will tell you to avoid it. Well, just like you do not have to give up your morning cup in pregnancy, you do not while breastfeeding either. In fact, it is so safe caffeine is sometimes given to premature infants in the NICU to help stimulate their breathing! Limit yourself to 200-300 mg per day, or 2 to 3 cups, per Infant Risk and the American Academy of Pediatrics (AAP). Watch your child's behaviors when you have ingested caffeine in order to assess how sensitive they are to it. Even though it is generally safe, some babies are too sensitive to it and get very fussy and overstimulated when their lactating parent has some coffee. There is also the risk of mild dehydration, as it is a diuretic, which can affect milk supply. Parents who are struggling with anxiety might want to avoid caffeine as well, as it can trigger physical symptoms similar to anxiety like higher cortisol, a panicked feeling, heart racing, and jitteriness. This can happen even with one cup, because just as each individual infant responds differently to caffeine, so too do adults.

Alcohol is another hot topic. Many say to just avoid it altogether. However, like with caffeine it is okay (with cautions) in moderation. The AAP recommends waiting until the baby is 2 months old to imbibe to allow for liver maturity, though other individual countries and world health authorities disagree that waiting is needed. If you personally feel uncomfortable you can pump your milk and dilute it with other milk later, save it in the freezer for when baby is older, or use it for milk baths. There is never a need to dump milk consumed while having an alcoholic beverage, as the content that goes into the milk is so low. The amount of alcohol in the milk increases and decreases as the amounts in the blood change. What is more dangerous about alcohol than the content in the milk is the ability to be able to care for the infant when intoxicated. It is best to have a sober caregiver available and avoid doing any co-sleeping on the nights you partake. Of importance is also that alcohol can reduce how efficiently the breast releases milk due to its effects on hormones, and the baby might nurse less due to the flavor changes; so even 1 glass comes with caution. While sometimes beer is reported to help with supply, it can end up having the opposite effect.

On the opposite end of the spectrum of total avoidance of alcohol is the camp that is overly encouraging of utilizing alcohol as a way to cope with the stresses of parenting. There are many people who subscribe to a culture that normalizes and encourages you to indulge to escape, and this can be very dangerous. It is a slippery slope to developing alcoholism when you start using alcohol to cope with the stressful days, because most of the days of early infancy and early childhood are very stressful. This is especially dangerous for parents who are already at risk for developing alcoholism or are suffering from postpartum mood disorders and seeking to self-medicate. Not only does this negatively impact your milk supply, but it can start to affect your parenting. Even if you avoid the risks of caretaking while under the influence of alcohol and are responsible enough to have a sober caretaker present at all times, alcohol affects your personality when you are sober. The regular consumption of alcohol depletes some vitamins that are key to our neurological, hormonal, and mood stabilization. It is likely to make you feel an exacerbation of the stress that you are trying to avoid and take you away from what could otherwise be quality time with your baby. High alcohol intake can alter baby's sleep patterns, cause poor weight gain, lead to hypoglycemia, or impair their motor development. So, as with coffee, be careful with alcohol. There are very good reasons that they are hot topics. Your babies deserve for you to take a good hard look in the mirror, and at them, to see how you are all affected by the consumption of these drugs, even in moderation. If you are struggling with safe and infrequent consumption then it might be time to seek help for controlling your alcohol intake.

Other drugs to consider are tobacco, marijuana and illicit or illegal drugs. Smoking, no matter the substance, introduces risks to you and to your baby. Second and third hand smoke expose the baby to toxins, and babies who are around smoke are at high risk for developing asthma, having frequent asthma attacks, having more frequent upper respiratory and ear infections, and have a higher risk of dying from SIDs than babies who are in non-smoking homes. Smoking not only introduces toxins but it alters the nutritional status of the milk. Ideally, no one in the house with a newborn will be smoking inside, and if they smoke outside then they should change clothes and wash their hands when they return. For now, we should assume the same for vaping until proven otherwise.

Drugs can also alter your ability to parent safely and can be passed through your milk to your baby. Some drugs if passed through the milk can result in infant death. Parents that do drugs are often investigated by child protective services, might be separated from their children, and are prohibited from breastfeeding, even when it is a legal drug in some states, like marijuana. There is not enough evidence to say that breastfeeding and doing any of these drugs is safe, and exposing children to them or causing them to ingest these drugs is illegal in most cases. Ideally, parents will be drug free while caring for their newborn. Marijuana is presently a gray area due to evolving legal changes and research developments, but most providers advise avoiding it due to lack of data on its safety during pregnancy and lactation.

If you are struggling with making good choices around drugs and alcohol, I have listed the contact for Substance Abuse and Mental Health Services Administration in my "resources" section, and that is a good place to start. You can also reach out to your healthcare team for help.

What is safe with food and drugs definitely changes if you have a baby who is premature or has certain health conditions, so consult your pediatrician and InfantRisk in those cases. Watch your baby and your self for signs of negative reactions to any food, drinks, or drugs that you ingest. Use your best judgement, consult professionals, and error on the side of caution when in doubt.

Breastfeeding and Sleep

Let us be honest, you do not get much sleep with a newborn regardless of feeding methods. If you are not aware of this yet, then you are grossly underprepared for parenthood. Normal sleeping and waking and eating habits of newborns do not vary much when you change their feeding methods. They have a drive to eat 8-12 times per day to encourage milk production. Changing the source of the milk does not over-ride their instincts. You will have many feeds back to back, and many throughout the night. It is developmental when their sleep habits change, and nothing to do with their food intake.

Babies sleep for more hours of the day than they are awake when newborns. This sleep is very broken up, so it does not usually seem like they are sleeping a lot, but they are. They will wake you frequently, day and night. Having interrupted sleep can be particularly challenging for new parents. In fact, interrupting sleep frequently has historically been used as a torture technique in some regions. My greatest suggestions to combat this are to manage your expectations, take turns feeding at night in two separate 6-hour shifts, and take a lot of naps.

To facilitate rest for a lactating parent, it is important to note that a lactating person can go 6 hours without nursing or pumping once in a 24 hour period without it dramatically impacting daily supply. Many parents like to take advantage of this by incorporating pumping and bottle feeding into their routine. The baby will likely still want or need to eat in that resting time, so a partner can give the baby pumped milk when it cues. Your lactation consultant can teach you alternate ways of feeding if you feel strongly about avoiding bottles. To replace the missed stimulation, the lactating person can pump an extra time early in the morning when they are most full due to higher prolactin, and take their turn resting in the early evening when it is at its lowest. That way the mammae might allow for the rest without waking them in pain from fullness, and they miss the pump and feeding sessions when output is the lowest. This also allows for a person to reach the typical goal of 8-12 feeding or pumping sessions per 24 hours. Sessions do not have to be a nice, neat every 2-3 hours and can be done with some sessions being back to back, much like how babies cluster feed.

My second suggestion for when the baby is in somewhat of a routine is to habitually go to sleep about 3 to 4 hours before you normally would, pre-baby. You will no longer get 6 to 8 hours of solid sleep, as it will be very interrupted. A good 10-12 hours of scattered and interrupted sleep feels a bit more restful. Combine this with the turn-taking at night, and it will save your sanity and your partnered relationship. We may not have our tribal villages, but we have our pumps and partners! We should utilize modern technology to our advantage. If you do not have a partner to help, enlist the help of another family member if you can.

Babies often like to be held while they are napping, so it helps to have other people around to take turns holding them. Babies napping on your chest is a common way to comfort your baby, let them get better sleep, and let them hear your heartbeat. You will need to be awake when they do this to monitor them, but it is not a problem and is normal for them to want to do this. It does not spoil them but teaches them that they can trust you and that they have a loving, nurturing, and responsive caregiver. Consistently meeting your baby's needs fosters independence because it helps them feel secure and safe. So, they do eventually outgrow this desire and start sleeping well in their own sleeping space.

You can adjust everyone's sleep schedule to the baby, even if that means everyone goes to bed at 7 pm, because that is when baby sleeps the longest. Additionally, implementing a "family nap time" where everyone in the house takes a midday nap when baby does can also help keep everyone well rested. Make sleep, and not chores, a priority the first few weeks. It is okay, everyone with a newborn has a house that looks like a tornado came through it.

As time goes on, babies do eventually sleep in longer stretches. After a few weeks, once per 24 hours you will get a 4 to 6 hour stretch, but sometimes it takes a few months to reach that milestone. Be prepared that some children wake every 2 to 3 hours for years. Yes, I do mean until they are 4 or 5 years old. This goes unchanged with changing feeding methods or adding more solids. Because, again, sleep is developmental and unrelated to food intake. They also go through sleep regressions, mental leaps, teething, and developmental milestones that tend to disrupt their sleeping patterns. If it seems you are past all those phases and your toddler does not get restful sleep regularly, and is having behavioral issues, they might need evaluation by a sleep or airway specialist to rule out any problems.

You will likely be tempted in your exhaustion to follow a sleep training method. You might also be erroneously advised by a well-meaning pediatrician that does not understand breastfeeding biological norms, that your baby should be sleeping more at their age or for longer stretches. They may advise sleep training when they should be referring you to an IBCLC to assess if the sleep pattern in relation to the breastfeeding relationship is normal.

Sleep training a breastfed baby is so challenging because many sleep consultants ruin breastfeeding relationships, and lactation consultants want you to martyr your sleep to nursing your baby. It is up to you to find a balance that you can live with. You might have to experiment with how your supply might handle longer stretches of sleep, as this causes some people's supply to dip, or the change cuts out too many feedings per day and causes baby to not get enough overall milk intake. I have seen sleep training take a baby from 8-10 feeds per day to 5 or 6, and because the lactating parent's capacity was only a few ounces at a time that cut out almost half of baby's daily calories. If you work with a sleep consultant, you need to simultaneously work with a lactation consultant to be sure it will not affect the baby or breastfeeding negatively. Even better, try to find someone who specializes in both sleep and lactation!

It is generally safe to encourage, but not force, good sleep habits. Encouraging baby to eat more frequently during the day may cut down on the number of nighttime feeds, as they meet their needs on a daily basis. Often, creating a womb-like sleeping space helps baby feel safe and sleep better. This would include having an extremely dark sleep space with a white noise like a fan whirring near the baby. Sometimes having something that smells like the parents near or in the sleeping space helps. To avoid creating a suffocation hazard, you might wrap a shirt the lactating parent has worn over the cot mattress. Warming the baby's bed before laying them in it helps, as well. Form fitting pajamas, swaddling, and sleep sacks help re-create the tight and snuggly feeling of being in the womb. Conversely, you would want a super bright and loud atmosphere during the day. These would all encourage good sleep hygiene without interfering with breastfeeding. Also, be alert that at 2-3 months of age babies will stop nursing to sleep at every feed during the day, and they will want to stay up and play. This does not mean they are not content, just that they are spending more time awake during the day, and are developmentally ready for more playtime.

Many parents find that breastfeeding and co-sleeping helps to keep them well-balanced. It can also promote more optimal breastfeeding as parent and baby are able to smell and hear each other all night, and the lactating parent can more closely identify and meet baby's needs. While the AAP recommends avoiding this, there is evidence contradicting that stance and it goes against the biological norms of the human species for the past tens of thousands of years.

Breast-sleeping is a term coined by Dr. James McKenna which describes a baby sleeping near a breast all night. He is a Ph. D. in biological anthropology who studies the biological norms and safety of lactating parents and babies sleeping together, while in a breastfeeding relationship. His website and books will answer all your questions about how to breast-sleep safely. His information is listed in the "resources" section.

Babies that at least sleep in the same room as their parents tend to nurse throughout the night which is greatly beneficial to over-all supply and infant safety. The feeding sessions between 12 and 5 AM are the most crucial to lactation success due to nightly hormonal signaling and fluctuations. It is also when lactating people s make the most milk, and thus baby gets the most milk. The frequent wakings are thought to be protective against SIDs (Sudden Infant Death Syndrome).

Co-sleeping might be baby in the same room, but it can also mean co-bedding like mentioned above. Even when most parents plan to avoid co-sleeping or co-bedding, they end up doing it anyway or on accident because they are desperate, and sleep deprived. If you have a safety plan, this can help you avoid making poor choices. When you are exhausted you might fall asleep with your baby in an unsafe space. Many suffocation accidents happen when a parent accidentally falls asleep with their infant in recliners and on couches.

The safest space for baby to sleep according to many experts is in their own cot or crib that has a firm mattress, no blankets, no pillows, no stuffed animals, nor bumpers, while lightly and snuggly dressed, and positioned on their back. This has been studied compared to other sleep arrangements and carries the lowest risk for baby. In addition, having babies sleeping in the same room the first 6 months of life, but not the same sleep space, reduces risks to baby. Babies do not typically like this arrangement and it triggers their instincts of fear of being alone, they know that being alone is dangerous, and they protest by crying or waking the moment you set them down. Dr. McKenna's research finds that when breast-sleeping, parent and baby sync in heart and breathing rates, both are more physiologically stable when bed sharing, and both get more restful sleep.

That being said, if you are going to sleep with your baby close to you there are some safety tips that should be followed, found through Dr. McKenna's research. Both adults that sleep in the bed must be light sleepers and not have taken any drugs or alcohol. Even better if it is just the lactating parent and the baby in the bed. Additionally, there should be no blankets or pillows in the bed. Parent and baby should be dressed warmly enough to not need them. Also, the bed should be firm and away from corners or walls, as baby can fall off the bed or fall into a gap and suffocate. Ideally, the bed would be in the middle of a room and the mattress on the floor. Baby still needs to be on their back, so the feeding parent should position themself such that they bring the breast to the baby who is positioned safely. There are many tips and images online on how to most safely co-bed together while breastfeeding. Dr. McKenna's book and website have the best information, and he conducts his research through the University of Notre Dame. Making the best decisions around sleep are another challenge of breastfeeding, and parenting.

Additionally, important to note, is that The Academy of Breastfeeding protocol for bedsharing concluded that "evidence does not support the conclusion that bedsharing among breastfeeding infants (i.e., breastsleeping) causes sudden infant death syndrome (SIDS) in the absence of known hazards." Their full statement is available to the public on their website.

It is biologically normal for infants to nurse to sleep, and there is no need to avoid doing this. It is also okay to seek other methods of soothing to sleep to involve other caregivers and give the lactating parent a break, but you should not feel forced to do so. The same is true for nursing toddlers, and sometimes after 1-3 years of night nursing parents decide to night wean because it is making life too difficult. As long as nutritional needs are being met, it is okay to be flexible with nursing to sleep. You will need to consider their nursing needs, developmental phase, and your own needs.

Another consideration that often comes up around night nursing is the health of the teeth. There are no valid studies that link night nursing to tooth decay, and breastfeeding can be protective against oral health issues. You can further reduce risks by having good oral hygiene. Tooth decay is often due to hereditary issues, poor oral hygiene, too many sugars or carbs in the solid diet, and imbalanced oral bacterial flora. There is no reason to avoid breastfeeding at night after teeth have erupted, but there might be issues with bottles. While the bottle may contain breastmilk, the issues are around the mechanics. When bottles are left with the baby, they might fall asleep with it in their mouth and then the milk is pooling in the mouth rather than being swallowed. When feeding on a breast the milk is aimed at the back of the mouth, past the teeth, and then swallowed. Pooling of milk happens less often when fed on the breast versus with a bottle. Best practice is not to leave the bottle with the baby in their sleep space, and to stop bottles at 1 year of age.

Sleep on formula versus breastfeeding is another thing to consider when making your choices about feeding and sleep. Formula is harder for babies to digest and some babies tend to sleep maybe 3 to 4 hours at a time rather than 2 to 3, and they seem to sleep more deeply. Many parents notice that if they give a formula bottle at night versus breastmilk, they get a longer stretch of sleep. As tempting as that is, it is actually over-riding protective benefits of breastfeeding and waking frequently. It also over-rides the baby's instincts to build and protect the milk supply. When a baby human feeds frequently and wakes frequently at night this is protective against Sudden Infant Death Syndrome (SIDS). As frustrating as this can be, it is what is best for your baby. It is also best for milk-supply to allow for those midnight feeds because of hormonal regulation of the supply, and certain hormones rising at night. If you are having to give formula, it is best to try to also provide some breast milk to help balance the risks.

Finally, on sleep, if no one has warned you I will take a moment here: babies routinely go through sleep regression phases, mental leaps, and teething. All of which will completely disrupt their sleep patterns. This is normal and developmental. Babies do not need to start eating solids at 4 months because they are waking more, although some people will try to convince you of this; the 4-month sleep regression is developmental and unrelated to solid food intake. When they are very close to mastering a new skill or understanding a more complex concept, they will have a mental leap and they sleep very poorly. This happens as they approach rolling over, crawling, pulling to stand, and walking. It also happens as their mind develops in complexity. They also sleep poorly when they are teething, which happens on and off for years. These are the times you will be tempted to get them to eat more to see if they will sleep better, and it will not work.

This brings us to our topic of introducing solids! It is a very exciting time, and many try to rush to it. It can even be a relief for a lactating parent to not be the only source of nutrition for baby. You have a lot to consider when starting solids, like when and what to feed! The most recent literature suggests that sometime between 4 to 6 months most children are ready to start solids. I believe the body does not lie and their little bodies tell us when they are ready. As I mentioned before, the sleep regression at 4 months is often mistaken as a sign of readiness, but it is not. Babies bodies signal they are ready for solids when they lose their tongue thrust reflex, they are able to sit up without assistance, and they have developed a pincher grasp.

The tongue thrust reflex is what helps them draw the breast deep into the mouth. If you tickle their mouth or chin, they should thrust their tongue out. This is often mistaken as a sign of hunger when caregivers touch their mouth and the baby sticks their tongue out, but they cannot help but exhibit this reflex when prompted. Much like the reflex in your knee to bring your leg shooting out when the doctor hits your knee just right. If they are tongue thrusting without being tickled, they are probably actually hungry. In order to draw food into the mouth and not just thrust it out and waste it, that reflex must stop happening. This reflex naturally goes away between 4 to 6 months.

Being able to sit up without assistance is important as it demonstrates that the baby has the core strength needed to cough out food if they gag or start to choke on it. Again, for most babies this strength develops between 4-6 months of age. They need plenty of opportunity to practice sitting up so they can develop the strength in their muscles. The sitting needs to happen without an aid, like an infant chair.

Finally, having developed a pincher grasp allows them to pinch and grab the food, and practice their hand-eye coordination by bringing the food to their mouth. Their body showing this sign of readiness is an important clue, just as the others are.

All of these signs should be present before offering solids, and you will also often see babies start reaching for food or staring at people who are eating around this time. Food before one is not just for fun, as is often touted. However, the volume of food actually swallowed does not need to be very much, as breastmilk or formula is their main source of nutrition for the first year. Food between 6 and 12 months is for developmental milestones, practice with hand eye coordination, and is an introduction to different flavors and textures. They need practice with foods to be able to successfully eat well after age one. It also helps prevent the development of food allergies when you introduce foods before one year of age. The most recent evidence suggests we should introduce high allergen foods to babies before their first birthday.

This is also the time that you can start offering water. Babies should not get water before solids are started due to the danger it poses to their organs. Formula and breastmilk contain enough hydration and the right balance of electrolytes. This is also why properly mixing formula is so important. Small amounts of water with solids are okay, and might help prevent constipation. The AAP suggests around 4 to 8 ounces of water per day are okay between 6 to 12 months of age, so you can try offering 1-2 ounces each time you offer solids. This will also help with practicing to use cups and straws, as the excitement of a new drink will encourage them to work towards using those items.

The only food you need to avoid the first year is honey, as their immune system is not ready to kill or destroy the botulism spores that might be present. This is true even of cooked honey, as heat does not destroy the spores. The only drink you need to avoid is any milk that is not formula or breastmilk. Dairy products can be introduced but other milks should not replace breastmilk or formula before they are 1 year old, as other milks do not have proper salt and fat content, which puts their kidneys and brain development at risk. It is also good practice to avoid sugary drinks like soda and juice, due to their connection to poor oral health and chronic disease development.

Nursing through chronic mental illness and trauma

Postpartum depression (PPD), postpartum anxiety (PPA), postpartum rage, postpartum psychosis, and other postpartum mood disorders can happen regardless of feeding method, however, having a challenging breastfeeding relationship makes you more likely to experience them. These can be compounded when a parent is overwhelmed with guilt because they feel like they are failing or not doing well. Parents are especially at risk if they are not getting adequate rest. If you experience this or start to feel that you are headed down this path due to breastfeeding challenges, please remember that your baby needs a happy and connected parent more than they need a full supply of breast-milk.

Many of a new parent's mental struggles come from not knowing whether the changes they are experiencing are normal or abnormal. Opening up this conversation and giving this brief education should serve to de-stigmatize some of these normal but scary changes, as well as de-stigmatize seeking help when it is warranted. Putting voice to these things removes the shame and creates safe spaces for parents to connect and open up.

One example of something that is normal, but upsetting, is how much we physically, mentally, and emotionally react to our infant crying. There is a deeply engrained biological call to action when an infant cries, and the intensity is exacerbated when it is an infant that we carried in our body and share genetic make-up with. Our body is meant to be sensitive to these cries, we are meant to want to do something to comfort them. It is like this to ensure that we will ensure that our offspring survive, and that their needs are met when they cry. Now, for some parents this feels extremely unsettling. It can feel like you want to crawl out of your skin, hop out a window, run away, or do something dramatic to make the feeling stop. Sometimes babies are inconsolable, and this can really grate our nerves. Feeling like this does not make you a bad parent, and having a baby that cries a lot does not make you a bad parent. This symbiotic relationship is designed to ensure bonding and survival, and the intensity is real and intentional. It is okay to need a break from this intensity or hand the crying baby to a different caregiver so you can go settle your nerves. When babies cry for hours and hours, as they sometimes do, you might need to go take a walk, send baby and partner for a walk, or set your baby in a safe space and go in a different room. If you need a few minutes with ear plugs in to dull the senses and internal responses, wear them. If you are making sure your baby is safe and cared for there is no reason to give power to or be ashamed about feeling overwhelmed when they cry.

Another completely normal part of taking care of a newborn is how the lack of sleep can affect you. You do not get much sleep when you have a newborn, less if breastfeeding does not go well, and even less when you are too upset to sleep because breastfeeding is not going well. Babies are very disruptive to sleep. In general, when we are exhausted we have a shorter fuse and we are more crabby than usual.

The highest risk factor for postpartum psychosis is lack of sleep, and it also lends to the development of all of the other mood disorders. It starts with exhaustion, which leads to delusions, and then there are hallucinations, which walks us into the psychosis. Prioritizing sleep is so important, and often not given enough attention or consideration when planning for the time frame when new parents are in the throes of newborn life. If you do not set yourself up to get some sleep, you will actually have a harder time falling asleep the more over-tired you are. If you do not sleep enough for several days in a row, you can have a psychotic episode and need hospitalized. This is almost always preventable. Work with your healthcare team and the people who are living with you to make a safe sleep-plan. If you find that you are unable to sleep, you need to tell your healthcare provider.

Another high risk-factor for postpartum mood disorders, especially depression, is being a female who has struggled with infertility. Parents who experience infertility often expect to hold onto their joy and elation every moment of the postpartum experience. This can feel very jarring and incongruent with the reality of being exhausted and overwhelmed by their newborn. Then there is the self-shame for feeling this, which leads to deeper and more consistent negative emotions. It is okay to not enjoy every moment or have moments of doubt and even negative feelings about having become a parent. At the same time we may go in and out of feeling high on the love we have for our infant. When we are sleep deprived and struggling, this push and pull is normal. This risk can be true of all parents, of course, but especially optimistic, and high-achieving personalities.

Common thoughts of parents who are struggling with mood imbalances are "Something has got to give," or "I don't feel like myself," or "I feel stuck," or "I am failing at this." You might experience suicidal thoughts, not feel connected to your baby, be overwhelmed easily, or feel you are a burden to your family. These can be clues that you might have PPD or PPA, and it is time to seek help.

Sometimes our PPD or PPA manifests as rage. You might find yourself losing control and yelling, even over minor things. You might struggle to tap into your patience, empathy, and logic. This is usually followed by a deep sense of regret and guilt, and leaves you wondering why you are lacking self-control with your anger. Often this can be a sign that you are taking on too much, and not honoring the postpartum rest and recovery that your body is needing. It can also mean you need to seek help with your PPD/PPA, with more logistical support, a healthcare assessment, counseling, or medications.

Some good news is that there is help available. You can

seek support groups, go to counseling, take herbs, take medications, or any combination of these options. Your team can help you find supportive resources for logistical things that are stressors, and help you work out what can be let go of temporarily to ease your burdens. They might also help you find the words and the courage to ask your loved ones for more help. Additionally, there are many safe medications, herbs, and treatments that can work well with breastfeeding. Plus, you have the option of utilizing a lactation consultant to address your breastfeeding challenges and worries head-on. If you are prone to mental illness or it runs in your family then it is a good idea to set up safety nets and support systems before you reach your postpartum period. Even parents with all the support in the world can still develop postpartum mood disorders, because it is largely hormonally driven. It is always wise to be realistic and prepare for the possibilities, regardless of risk factors.

I do not even particularly like the term mood disorders, because it sets us up to blame it on being in the wrong mood or a bad mood. Really, the body is struggling to produce the right neurochemicals in the brain, like serotonin and dopamine, which both produce happy feelings. Sometimes, medication is needed when our body is not making enough of something. This is true with mental health and many other issues in the body. Some examples are taking iron when you are anemic, taking thyroid replacement when you have hypothyroidism, or taking insulin when your pancreas stops producing it and you are diabetic. Many parts of our body get dysfunctional from time to time, and none of us make it to old age without at least one body part needing some help. Parents who acknowledge they are struggling with this are often successful with breastfeeding because they get the tools they need to cope and to correct the hormonal and neurochemical imbalances. There are many safe medication options for postpartum neurochemical imbalances that are causing symptoms of depression and anxiety.

If you experience postpartum psychosis or are admitted to the hospital due to severe mental health concerns, you may be put on medications that make your milk temporarily unsafe for baby. However, you can still pump to continue the milk supply. It is ok to ask for the tools and help to do this while inpatient. Save all of your pumped milk until discharge, and then look up all your medications to make sure the milk is safe before feeding it to baby. If it is definitely not safe you can then dump that milk, but then resume nursing or pumping as normal. Even if you are unable to keep up with the pumping, it is possible to re-lactate or return to breastfeeding after an interruption or separation such as this.

It is partially expected and normal to have heightened anxiety or a state of constantly worrying about your baby. Biologically, you are designed to be the protector of this offspring. Your brain wants you to worry about them! This can (and often does) present as intrusive scary thoughts, like suddenly worrying about car accidents, drownings, or harm coming to the baby. Knowing this surge of worrying is normal often keeps you from going down the path of worrying about how much you are worrying. There is also a component of this that makes it hard to accept help, even from our partner. There is a deep fear they do not and will not take care of your baby to the standards you have set internally. There is an unspoken expectation that you should just know how to do this and be able to do it alone. For your mental health, you need to trust other caregivers to give you a break. We are just not designed to take care of newborns alone.

Our exhaustion also makes us edgy and negative. You may resent your baby when they wake more than usual at night. You also might resent your partner for sleeping through midnight feeds. Often when we are tired, we are snappier and more emotional. The body and the soul are under a lot of pressure, often self-imposed. Learning to adjust and grow with these big changes is really hard, and its ok to have these feelings and have a hard time.

Another symptom of our exhaustion and overwhelm might be fantasizing about leaving our family and moving away to be single and alone. We may find ourselves jealous of childless friends. Our thoughts wandering there and imagining that different life are just thoughts, they are not an actual plan. People often daydream about a different life when they are feeling unhappy, and just because you are in love with your baby and partner does not mean you will always avoid feeling unhappy all of the time. If you are struggling with getting enough support or rest, you might start feeling burnt out and want to escape. Avoiding negative feelings is a natural way of coping with them, and most people engage in daydreaming about alternative realities when they are feeling down. You might do this at work or in school, and it just feels heavier when you do it at home, but it is not any more serious. It can be another way that our body is communicating with us that it needs something. This might be your internal white flag being raised, calling out for help and peace.

Your brain changes and remaps many connections in order to adjust to being a caretaker to an infant. It helps us to connect with and protect our children, but it is not without its downsides. It can present like anxiety and grief, and like what many call "mom brain." The brain is sleep deprived and remarkably busy in a way that it has never been. This feels overwhelming and strange the first time you experience it, but it is largely normal. A great change is needed in ourselves in order to adjust to our new roles. This shift can also happen in the other caretaker or parent, and often does, just as postpartum depression and anxiety can happen in them as well.

When a parent has a challenging or traumatic pregnancy or labor experience it can interfere with being able to bond with the infant during pregnancy, and the parent may not feel a super strong connection immediately. When a parent had a traumatic or neglectful childhood, they may need years of interaction with their child before feeling deeply connected to them. There are many variations of normal with our attachment and bonding to our children, and sometimes that even varies from child to child. Even without trauma, not every parent feels immediately intensely bonded to their offspring. Some people find the hormonal boosts of nursing help to forge this connection. Skin to skin can help boost the bonding hormones when nursing is not an option. There is no need to feel guilty for the variations of normal, but many people do. This can inhibit normal biological responses to the infant, and sometimes you will have to override your brain and emotional responses and just power through the motions. You might feel like you are faking it until you make it, and this is especially true of parents with mood disorders but can affect all parents.

Sometimes the changes in the first few weeks postpartum present as "baby blues" which is like a mild depression or moodiness. This can be hard when you are expecting to feel mostly joyous, and then are confronted with negative emotions and exhaustion. You might feel sad sometimes, without a reason. You might cry unexpectedly, for a good reason, for a bad reason, or for no reason. There is no right way to feel postpartum, every person experiences these changes differently. They can be different with each pregnancy, as well. It will be important to allow yourself some grace in the time period.

These moods and emotions are largely linked to the huge hormonal changes. We have a boost in prolactin that in-turn decreases dopamine. Prolactin is needed to build supply. Dopamine is responsible for our sense of happiness. The hormones progesterone and estrogen are also high during pregnancy and contribute to creating more dopamine and serotonin, and they rapidly decline right after delivery. So, the hormones run the show; not our logic, nor attempts at self-regulation. Some parents find omega fish-oil and magnesium supplements to be helpful in this time, as the healthy fats and magnesium play a large role in our neuro-receptor and hormone health. If these negative feelings stick around for more than a couple of weeks or get progressively worse, it will be time to talk to your doctor about postpartum depression.

Postpartum depression is similar to other depression conditions and is diagnosed based on its relativeness to being in a postpartum state. You can develop postpartum depression at any time in the first 2 years of your child's life. You are also subject to developing a very similar condition called weaning depression, which we discuss more later on in the book. When depressed you may experience physical discomfort, sadness, an urge to cry, loss of enjoyment of foods and hobbies, difficulty sleeping, wanting to sleep more than usual, feeling unmotivated, and lacking the energy or motivation to maintain usual hygiene habits. Postpartum depression can also present as anger, rage, or obsessive intrusive thoughts. Sometimes depression can cause you to think of hurting yourself or your baby, and this does not make you a bad parent. Your healthcare team knows that if you admit to these scary thoughts, it is because you desperately want to avoid acting on them. The help you need is available, all you need to do is make it clear that you want it. This will not put you at risk of child services taking your child, they are almost never called or consulted just because a parent admits these thoughts, especially in the absence of a formulated plan.

A majority of parents actually report having particularly scary intrusive thoughts, so scary thoughts are not unique to the condition of postpartum depression or anxiety. Intrusive thoughts happen so often and to most parents, so they are not technically a mood disorder. They are also not an intention to act and might be a subconscious way our mind reminds us to all the dangers we must consider for our offspring. Intrusive thoughts are usually very disturbing and very upsetting, yet most parents experience them. They can include thoughts of extreme harm coming to you or your baby, sexual thoughts about your baby, a flashing image of hurting yourself or your baby, and illogical scenarios like sharp objects that are far away in a safe space being able to cut your baby. When they are fleeting and random, you can manage them well.

When you move beyond being able to cope with them, they are persistent, or they keep you from achieving tasks then they might be triggering an obsessive-compulsive disorder. If they are interfering with your daily life or you feel you are not coping with them well then it is time to seek help. An example might be avoiding breastfeeding for fear of smothering the baby, no matter how unlikely. Another example of not coping well might be avoiding caring for your baby because you think the scary and intrusive thoughts make you an unsafe caregiver. Remember to just label them as only thoughts, acknowledge them, allow them to pass, and do not give them power over you. Know they may happen again and are not a reflection of an intention or a magical premonition. Do not try to avoid the thoughts, and do not dwell on them. They are not a reflection of your true self, or your plans. If the scary thoughts are truly concerning you or overwhelming you, then you can work with a mental health professional on how to cope.

In the same arena as mental health is avoiding overstimulation. Overstimulation can be a sensory challenge for those of us who are sensitive to so much interaction, noise, and touching. Couple that with stimulation from a spouse and other children, and things get overwhelming quickly. This can be due to a low stimulation threshold, sensory processing disorders, anxiety, or a trauma response.

Even without previous issues many parents find themselves feeling "touched out" especially when being in close physical high-touch interaction with an infant and older children for most hours of the day. This often presents as irritability, so if you feel crabby try taking some time alone. Many parents are shocked when they find how angry and irritable they become. It is okay to ask for a break and step away! When your body is reacting with rage, aversion, or extreme sadness, it is trying to tell you it needs something.

Another way that breastfeeding can connect us to or bring up the past is with our history of sexual experiences, especially if we have a history of being sexually abused. Something many healthcare providers will skim over asking about is if you have ever experienced sexual abuse or trauma. This can be especially important to your breastfeeding relationship and mental health during this time in your life, as your delivery and breastfeeding will involve making your body accessible and vulnerable to not only your baby, but many healthcare workers. While breastfeeding itself is not sexual, is still involves what is sometimes an erogenous zone utilized in sexual experiences—the mammae.

We cannot help that our body triggers certain hormones when breastfeeding, one being oxytocin. Oxytocin is what makes breastfeeding a pleasant, loving, and bonding experience. This is the same hormone that boosts during labor when the uterus contracts, and tugs on the cervix. This is the same hormone that boosts to deliver the placenta. This is the same hormone that boosts when a baby nurses to help contract and shrink the uterus back to its nonpregnant size. This is the same hormone that boosts during orgasm to stimulate motion in the cervix to draw semen into the uterus, and helps us bond with our lover.

Breastfeeding is meant to be pleasurable, were it not we would not have survived very long as a species. It is by no accident that oxytocin, a hormone of pleasure, is linked to the act of breastfeeding. Sexual pleasure and breastfeeding being pleasurable both promote our survival as a species. It is important to make the distinction between general pleasure, and sexual pleasure. Our body cannot always distinctly differentiate these, especially when they are triggered by the same hormonal cascade, but our logical mind can learn to differentiate them. Knowing that oxytocin surges during orgasms, breastfeeding, and labor can help you make sense of what your body is feeling without having to feel ashamed or scared of natural bodily functions.

Even when you understand this, the physical challenges of the logistics of a nursing relationship can generate negative feelings. Often feeling "trapped" while nursing for hours on the couch while having your nipples suckled can be extremely triggering for survivors of sexual abuse, especially if the abuse involved feeling trapped or having the nipples touched. On the other hand, some have the opposite response and find it very healing to use their mammae the way nature intended, and it helps them remove the sexual association.

Perhaps you will find you react with a combination of both, and other big feelings. Just know to be prepared for intense feelings about breastfeeding if you are a survivor of sexual abuse or assault. Make time to sit with your emotions around it. Give yourself some grace and compassion, and time to work through it. It might be a good idea to seek counseling around the idea beforehand, so that you go into the process prepared and with some tools to handle the big feelings.

Even without a history of being sexually assaulted or abused the feelings in your body created from hormones during breastfeeding are strange and difficult to distinguish from sexual pleasure or arousal at times for some, due to the oxytocin surges. This can feel scary or off-putting and may make you question if how you are feeling is normal or acceptable. The thing is breastfeeding had to be pleasurable or parents would not continue long enough to optimize their baby's growth the first few years of life when they could not eat solid foods or had scarce amounts of food. The intense pleasure and bond had to be formed in order to ensure that the female parent would continue to offer the breast and stay close to the infant, despite how hard and exhausting it was to care for them. Try to view your body, and this nursing relationship, outside of the lens of your life in this modern lifestyle; and consider the design and its survival advantages to the species over thousands of years. If it is still too much to handle for you, it is okay to choose not to breastfeed.

Additionally, parents who face extremely challenging nursing relationships in the beginning often feel traumatized and easily triggered to fear, panic, or depression when issues surface, and it can be hard to move forward with breastfeeding progression. Many people carry their heavy feelings around breastfeeding not going well for years. Those feelings are valid and understandable, and it is ok to seek help working through them and to take longer to get comfortable with breastfeeding after the initial trauma has passed. Sometimes progressing breastfeeding is just as much about mental health as it is about a lactating person's and baby's physical capability. It might take time to learn to trust your body. This can also be true following infertility, a difficult pregnancy, or a traumatic labor and delivery process.

While help is definitely available for struggles with our emotional health, many often find they are dismissed or not taken seriously when they attempt to ask for help. Though unfair, you might have to be very clear and assertive with your expectation for more support and mental health resources if you feel your maternal healthcare team is not grasping how un-well you feel. When people around you dismiss your negative emotions or try to focus on only positive things, this is called toxic positivity. Generally, this has more to do with the other person being uncomfortable with allowing others to be upset than it does with the validity of your feelings. It is okay to look for a safe space to be upset; you can ask that your feelings not be dismissed, and ask that they not try to fix it. Sometimes support and expressing ourselves is all we need. It will be important to setting up your mental health support for when baby is here to make sure you have 1 or 2 people that will be this safe space for you. This might be a therapist, your partner, a family member, or a friend.

It is important to note that everything I just reviewed is also subject to consideration for the other parent of your newborn. Fathers or other parents might experience postpartum mood disorders, have posttraumatic stress that influences their parenting, have a history of sexual abuse that influences how they feel about breastfeeding, or just generally struggle with all the changes that being a new parent brings.

Nursing through illnesses

Many parents believe, or are erroneously advised, that they cannot nurse a baby if they are ill. No short-term illness requires that you wean, or temporarily stop nursing. The greatest risk is temporary supply reduction and dehydration to you and your baby. The safest course of action is to drink extra electrolyte preparations, and watch baby's diaper count. A good source of electrolytes might be an electrolyte drink or water with a pinch of salt added. Commercial electrolyte sports drinks often have more sugar than electrolyte content. Find a low sugar electrolyte drink to keep in the cupboard for when you need it. Monitor baby's diaper output, if it gets low then supplement temporarily. Always work with healthcare professionals to make sure you and baby are stable enough to keep breastfeeding without supplementation, and that any medications you might need are safe for your baby and will not affect your supply. Common upper respiratory illness remedies like menthol in cough drops and pseudoephedrine can cause a supply dip.

It is important to practice precautions when ill, to try to avoid getting baby sick. Though they are protected due to an immune response with exposure to the antibodies through breastmilk, it is always best to avoid the illness if possible. Washing your hands frequently helps, but especially before handling the baby or anything you feed the baby with such as your pumping equipment or bottles. A mask might be worn if you have an upper respiratory illness to prevent coughing and sneezing too close to the baby. Skin to skin is also beneficial to boosting the immune system for both the parent and the baby. While the thought of passing an illness to your infant is scary, general precautions are more than enough.

When your baby is ill, it is still best to nurse on demand. Even if baby is throwing up, nursing as much as baby is willing will help keep them hydrated. Nursing on demand is especially important with diarrhea, and breastmilk alone is usually enough for mild stomach bugs. If your baby has low diaper counts, they may need extra hydration. You might have to get them to sip on expressed milk in small quantities or breastfeed every few minutes. In extreme cases, babies might need intravenous hydration, and nursing will help comfort them through that. When babies have colds, you might have to keep them upright or relieve their nasal congestion with saline, breastmilk, steamy showers, or cool mist humidifiers. If they are unable to breastfeed due to their cold symptoms, you may have to temporarily pump and bottle feed to ensure adequate hydration and to protect your milk supply.

Chronic illness can be different, especially if it is an illness or disease that has a need for medications that can be passed through breast milk. Some chronic illness can be nursed through or even suppressed by nursing. The list of medications required for chronic illnesses that may make nursing unsafe is short. Some chronic infections like infectious hepatitis and AIDs can be passed through the breastmilk, and depending on the disease the risk might outweigh the benefit. It would also be weighed with your ability to access clean water and formula. It would be best to work with your healthcare team to make a plan around if breastfeeding needs to be partial, or if it is safest not to breastfeed.

Chronic illness or disease in babies might make them too weak to nurse, or unable to digest breastmilk. You might have to pump and bottle feed or give special formula. If your baby has something that they might give to you through skin contact, you might have to pump.

Breastfeeding through personal emergencies, natural disasters, power outages, pandemics, war, and times of famine presents its own challenges. The over-all recommendation would be to continue to nurse because the breast milk will provide antibodies, nutrition, and hydration.

Food and water might be scarce in times of uncertainty, and breastmilk can be a continued source of comfort and help meet baby's nutritional and hydration needs. As long as a lactating person has water, they can continue to produce the milk from the water, fat stores, and stores of nutrients in the bones. They will contain all the ingredients needed to make the milk. If a parent is exposed to a viral or bacterial source of infection during an emergency, then the milk will provide antibodies to the baby. Though, war, pandemics, and natural disasters do make the logistics of breastfeeding support more challenging as resources are pulled or re-allocated to other causes.

Even with a parent needing a surgery, continuing on their milk is still the best option. You should be given access to a pump if you have surgery and are lactating. Most parents will be told to dump their milk, but this is almost never necessary, especially if you request that nursing friendly medications be used. Some common examples of surgeries needed postpartum might be gallbladder removal, hemorrhoid correction, placenta removal, or hematoma resolution. After surgery as soon as you are coherent it is safe to pump or nurse. After surgery if you have intense itching due to reactions to medications then you will want to avoid antihistamine as it might dry you up. You can safely use calamine lotion or hydrocortisone cream to relieve your symptoms.

In emergencies, it is logistically easier to access a female's milk, even with pumping, than it is to have everything you need to continue to safely formula feed. It would not be unheard of for a breastfeeding parent to share the milk with other family members to help protect or hydrate them in emergencies, as well. It is wise to have emergency and contingency plans, such as a manual pump that does not need power, the knowledge of how to hand-express, and backup formula and clean water, just in case.

Assume everything goes pretty well

Okay let us assume you are capable of nursing 5 children for 4 years each, with abundant supply, no latch pain, no infections, and everything is basically perfect. It is still hard. You really cannot ever expect everything to go perfectly. You will be faced with what seems like infinite decisions and options, and often in healthcare those decisions are made for you. Challenges during this time are inevitable.

What can be challenging might be the abrupt change in lifestyle and demand that is placed on the nursing parent. Additionally, how these changes affect your relationship and your partner. Cluster feeding, leaking, lack of sleep, growth spurts, teething, engorgement, and being the primary caretaker are just some of those challenges and the challenges begin right away.

Another example is that when breastfeeding or pumping, you will also experience "after pains" or essentially, more contractions. Each time the baby nurses the first few days the hormone oxytocin is triggered to keep contracting the uterus back down to its smaller original size, as well as to release the milk. With each cramp or contraction, you may feel a gush of blood come out. Sadly, after-pains tend to get worse and stronger with each baby. Nurses in the hospital also tend to want to massage your uterus to make sure it is firming up and you are not at risk of hemorrhaging, which is triggering to an after-pain episode. You will also need to urinate and emptying the bladder will bring on the pains again. If you cannot urinate, you might have to get a temporary catheter, for a few hours to a few days, because they will not risk bladder rupture and the urethra might be too swollen to allow urine to pass through. It can be hard to concentrate on nursing when so many other things are going on with your body.

All of the decisions you will face in labor and delivery will be a challenge, too. Things as simple as deciding when to bathe, or if to bathe, your baby will come into question. Some argue the smell and the vernix on the baby should not be washed away, as they emit pheromones that help the parent's brain recognize, bond with, and make milk for the baby. There are studies that support this.

You will be faced with decisions around labor options, pain management, vaccines, vitamins, skin care, when to cut or clamp the umbilical cord, what to do with the placenta, who to have present at delivery, who will you allow to visit the newborn, and many more choices. There is so much to learn and so many things to decide, and sometimes your decisions will be challenged in the moment, especially in emergencies.

Managing your expectations is key to making this time easier on you, and your partner. Knowing what to expect as normal and being prepared for challenges will help you relax and feel confident in your parenting. Even when not breastfeeding, thinking of the first 3 months postpartum as the "fourth trimester" where parent and baby are one unit will help you wrap your head around how much the baby physically needs you. They need frequent feeding and holding, as well as responsive parents in order to feel safe, loved, nurtured, and nourished. Their needs are more than physical. As you meet their calls to action with a physical response you are also nurturing their psychological and emotional health.

You will need to hope for the best but prepare for the worst. Anticipate that things may not go as planned. Your labor and delivery may be unexpected or traumatic. Those around you that you place your trust in might betray that trust or coerce you into decisions that they think are best but contradict your plans. It will be critical to have a support person present to help ask questions and promote your wishes. Preparing for labor and delivery possibilities is part of preparing to breastfeed, as many things that happen in that time influence breastfeeding relationships. You might need to work through some anxiety, depression, and grief from birth trauma, if you experience it, in order to be able to connect better with yourself and your baby.

You will want to generally familiarize yourself with normal baby behaviors and bodily functions. For breastfeeding you will want to learn about the let-down, suckling, non-nutritive suckling, and the suck-swallow-breathe pattern. It is normal behavior for babies to need to suckle frequently, cry a lot, wake frequently, spit up a lot, poop a lot, have very thin poop, and have a lot of gas. Gas is a huge concern for most new parents because it seems to upset the babies and happen often. Safe remedies like probiotics, gripe water, tummy massage, and bicycle legs might help, but knowing how normal it is might keep you from chasing the perfect remedy for weeks. You should definitely keep outfit changes handy for the baby as well as caretakers, because the spit up and poop might end up all over your clothes.

They also make a lot of very strange noises that do not sound like normal breathing, and they hiccup frequently. They might grunt or groan, or cycle through more rapid breathing episodes. They also might jerk their bodies suddenly while falling asleep or changing positions, or shake their limbs a bit. Being unfamiliar with newborn noises and behaviors often causes parents to needlessly worry. When in doubt, take a video or picture and show it to your healthcare provider to confirm if it is normal or not. Call emergency services if the strange noises are accompanied by rib retractions, or the baby's mouth or face turning blue.

To combat worries around your baby's milk intake, it helps to know how much you should be expecting them to eat. Expected milk intake is very small the first few days, and there are excellent graphics you can keep at hand if needed. Every day the first 1-2 weeks the amount needed at each feeding increases at a dramatic rate. They often want to nurse frequently, even when they are getting enough volume. We expect that babies take at each feed 5-15 ml of milk by day 2, 15 to 30 ml by day 3, 30 to 45 ml by day 4, 45 to 60 ml by day 5, and most babies take

75-90 ml by day 7. The increase is less dramatic between days 7 to 14. Most infants want 80 to 100 ml by 2 to 3 weeks of age and anywhere between 80 to 150 ml by 1 month. The appetite and metabolic needs of the baby combined with the capacity of the mammae will determine the long-term feeding volumes. If baby is just at breast, you do not need to know the exact amount the baby is drinking—just monitor diaper output, as it reflects adequate intake. Your healthcare providers will typically monitor the weight gain, as well. If there is a question of adequate intake, you can seek what is called a "weighted feed" with a professional. This involves weighing the baby, feeding the baby, and then weighing again to get an approximation of how much milk the baby transferred from the breast to their stomach. You should bring the baby hungry to these appointments. If you are bottle feeding or assessing transfers it helps to know these numbers. Expected intake after the first few weeks is usually 20-30 ounces per day, 24-26 ounces per day being average (about 1 oz per hour). The daily average is stable from about 1 month to 6 months of age. At six months it might decrease, not increase, as solids start to be part of the diet. Of course, there are always babies outside of the averages. It is best to get a professional assessment because they can evaluate the health of the infant to determine if they are thriving, outside of normal intake or not. There are many other things to measure and assess aside from weights and diaper counts.

It is important to note that most lactating people do not need to be able to pump 5-10 ounces per session like the many parents you see on social media with over supply! Families usually do not need a large freezer stash, and a small one is sufficient for emergencies. It is best to try not to obsess over numbers of milliliters or number of ounces. For most parents, the focus should be on feeding the baby, not stocking the freezer. The stress of obsession is never good for milk production, anyhow. In fact, the rise of cortisol with stress often lowers supply.

As I mentioned, the numbers you do want to watch and closely monitor are diaper output and periodic weight checks.

Someone should weigh the baby daily or every other day the first week, then weekly the first 2-3 weeks, and every 2-3 months after that. This will happen at your child's well-checks with the pediatrician and if you are working with an IBCLC. Weight might be checked more often early on as you work out breastfeeding troubleshooting.

Diaper count is an excellent indicator of intake because it reflects adequate hydration. Physically, we must have good fluid intake in order to have adequate fluid output. We hope that a baby has 1 wet and 1 stool diaper on the first day of life. This is usually fluid and particles from the baby swallowing amniotic fluid. The first stool is meconium, which is a thick, sticky, black and tar-like stool. On days 2-3 the fluid urine output and stool are made up of a combination of swallowed colostrum and the previously swallowed amniotic fluid. There should be at minimum 2 wet diapers and 1-2 stools on day 2, and 3 wet diapers and 2-3 stools on day 3. Sometimes babies have what is called "brick dust" urine that looks like a thick salmon colored deposit in the diaper. This is a common sign that dehydration is starting to occur or has occurred in the last few days. As long as they do not persist past day 3-5, there are other signs of adequate hydration, and there is not more than a few of them, it is likely harmless. As the milk starts to come in days 3-5, we see more changes in the diapers. Usually the stool slowly transitions from thick meconium to a thin curdy or seedy yellow. While it is transitional you may see meconium and a mix of textures and colors like greens, yellows, and oranges mixed in. Usually a minimum of 4 wet diapers and 1-3 stools on day 4, then 5 wet diapers and 1-3 stools on day 5, and 6 wet diapers and 1-3 stools on day 6. Keep in mind these are minimums and not an indication baby is getting enough milk to thrive, but only enough to be well hydrated. Weight gain will tell us if the intake is adequate. Most babies will have more diapers than the minimum, once milk comes in. Many providers will ask you about diaper count the first few weeks, so keep a detailed log.

Weight loss and weight gain of the infant will be discussed

frequently the first few weeks of life. We expect babies to lose up to 10% of their birth weight within the first few days of life. As they await the mature milk, they are also re-balancing the fluids in their bodies. They are often swollen from being in-utero, especially if you received a lot of extra intravenous fluids during labor. Many practitioners argue that if a laboring person got extra fluids for induction, epidural, or cesarean, then the infant's birth weight is slightly inflated. This might mean we are able to be more flexible on the 10% weight loss expectation, but it will also depend on diaper count and other data. Baby's burn their fat more easily than adults, so the babies burn fat off while they wait for the mature milk. This is because baby's have special easy to access brown fat, while adults have a more stubborn yellow fat. They also have a belly full of amniotic fluid that they had been swallowing when they were practicing suckling and swallowing in utero. So, most babies tolerate this weight loss well.

When a baby loses 10% and is not having enough diapers, this is often when supplementation is suggested. It is important to make a plan and not ignore this suggestion. Supplementation can be your own pumped milk, or donor milk if it is available, or formula. The reason we use this as a barometer is because studies have shown us that at this level of weight loss babies start to become high risk for other complications. Complications might be hypoglycemia, jaundice, poor body temperature stability, dehydration, and sometimes even seizures if the dehydration and hypoglycemia are low enough. If it feels like the medical team is trying to scare you into supplementing, they might be. We do not suggest supplementing to make our lives easier, we do it to keep the baby safe and healthy. So, if you face this, remember that it is time to consult the IBCLC and make a plan that not only protects the baby, but also protects your supply and the breastfeeding relationship. Being prepared for this possibility is only realistic, as a majority of first-time parents need to supplement the first week of their baby's life. Additionally, studies show that supplementation with proper support leads to better long-term breastfeeding success rates, so do not be afraid of it.

Ranges of normal for feeding frequency can be a big clue to whether or not baby is getting enough to eat, so be sure to note down somewhere how long and how often your baby is nursing. Babies tend to nurse every 10 to 20 minutes during cluster-feeding sessions, or sometimes every hour, then most feeds are every 2 to 3 hours, and sometimes they are nice to you and give you a long stretch of 4 to 6 hours for sleeping. Babies should generally not sleep for 4 to 6 hour stretches until they are past their birth weight and around 2 weeks old. You might get permission from a healthcare provider to allow this to happen sooner than 2 weeks if things are going exceptionally well. One long stretch of sleep every 24 hours allows the baby's growth hormone to boost, and this is helpful to optimal development. They will want to feed about 8-12 times in 24 hours, but this is usually not a neat every 2 to 3 hour pattern. Frequent feeding does not mean they are not satisfied, and they will cluster feed even when their stomach is very full. This is ingrained and instinctive behavior that encourages the milk supply to keep increasing the first 4 to 6 weeks, and sometimes precedes a longer stretch of sleep. Cluster feeding tends to happen in the early evening when supply dips and babies are over-tired and over-stimulated from a long day. The milk is fattier when there is lower volume and might help the baby sleep a longer stretch after the evening cluster session. Cluster feeding may also happen between midnight and five in the morning due to the abundance of milk flow and baby's instincts to night-feed. This helps them get large volumes of milk and it serves to stimulate the daily prolactin amounts, and thus overall daily milk production.

As the baby gets older, they will change their patterns. This is especially true when they are ready to drop a nap every few months, and the feeding pattern will adjust. This is a time many parents worry about the supply changing, and there is no need. The body will adjust to the baby's new schedule. How frequently your older infant nurses will depend on your capacity. Mammae that can hold 2-3 ounces at a time will often correspond with a baby that continues to nurse 8 times in 24 hours.

Breasts that have a larger capacity might correspond with a baby nursing only 6 times in 24 hours, because they are drinking a larger quantity less often. For example, 5-6 ounces at a time 6 times per 24 hours. This will also depend on how well they take to solids.

The amount of time a baby nurses varies quite a bit in the beginning. Feedings may range from 5 to 60 minutes in the first few weeks. Expect to see a suck-swallow-breathe pattern that makes it appear that they are taking a break from nursing for a moment. If a lactating person has an extremely fast flow and the baby is very efficient, time at the breast can be 5 to 10 minutes on each breast and done! Some people have slower flows, and some babies are slower to eat so they take maybe 20 to 30 minutes on each breast. Most babies generally become more efficient with time. It is only concerning if a baby is eating for exceptionally long periods and still not content after most feedings. If it is unclear to you if the behavior is normal or not, then seek professional assessment and guidance.

It is also helpful to know about early feeding cues. The baby's body gives many clues that it is ready to suckle, even before they start crying. It may be as subtle as opening and closing the mouth frequently. Sometimes they stick their tongue out repeatedly, or turn their heads in search of the nipple, or rooting. When very young, they might bring their hands to their mouth, but this is a short-lived cue because they very soon start discovering and chewing on their hands for fun. They may start making humming noises or start bobbing their head up and down like a chicken pecking for food. They may lick their lips, stretch, and increase their movement. Usually, crying is the last cue. Then, you will need to help them calm down before offering the breast, so start with skin to skin and talking to them in a soothing voice.

Breastfeeding is a new skill to you and to your baby. With each new baby you will learn new things. Parenting the first time is going to require the development of many new skills, and your hands will be clumsy as you learn to hold and move and care for the tiny fragile baby. Most parents will fear handling a newborn; you will not know the feeling of changing diapers, your hands will feel awkward as you practice a deep latch, and you will feel strange as you learn how exactly to burp them. These skills come with time and practice. The more you do them, the better you become. Humans are not born knowing these motor skills, like many other mammals; they must be practiced in order to be perfected. Do not compare yourself to the consultant, practitioner, or nurse who has handled hundreds if not thousands of newborns.

It is never wrong to feed a hungry baby if you are unsure if your baby is getting enough. Just be sure to have a professional assess breastfeeding as soon as possible if you are feeling like you need to supplement. Supplementing when it is not needed will ultimately sabotage the breastfeeding relationship. It becomes a self-fulfilling prophecy as you continue to offer more supplement, your supply will decrease due to reduced breast stimulation. If you are needing to supplement due to low supply, you will need help balancing the breast and bottle in a way that maximizes your supply.

You will also need to manage expectations about how you will handle being a parent. You might plan to do things a certain way and change your mind in the moment or as you learn more. Being flexible with expectations versus reality is a helpful mental health tool that enables us to be more resilient when we face challenges. This can be helpful with little things and big things. A little thing might be planning to use a clip to identify which breast you last nursed on versus the reality of just groping your breast to feel which one is most full. Big things might be planning to avoid going in public the first 3 months of baby's life, versus the reality of missing social interaction at the store, or the act of shopping itself. Try to remain flexible, and keep your sense of humor!

Deciding How Long to Breastfeed

Another stressor around breastfeeding can be deciding how many months or years to breastfeed for, if at all. If child and parent so desire the relationship can go on indefinitely. There are current and historical instances of children nursing past the age of 10 years. In some communities the longer you nurse the stronger your child is perceived to become. Breast milk can be beneficial to us no matter our age, given the make-up of what human milk is.

The World Health Organization recommends nursing for 2 years and beyond, as long as both the parent and the baby (or child) are interested and happy with the relationship. The first 6 months will ideally be only breastmilk or formula. Many toddlers lose interest as they take on more solids and become busier, but some will nurse for years as they continue to enjoy the milk and the closeness with and comfort from their parent. The American Academy of Pediatrics recommends at least 1 year, with the first 6 months being exclusively breastmilk or formula.

Biologically, anatomically, and anthropologically it is ideal to nurse until about 3-4 years old. Our thymus gland, which sets up our lifetime immunity strength, develops until we are 3-4 years old. The thymus is larger in breastfed infants, suggesting breastmilk passes considerable chronic immunity protection. Then starting around age 5, our "milk teeth" start falling out. Our smaller "milk teeth" start falling out when we are ready for heartier and harder to eat foods and have stronger jaws to enable this. Children without cultural constraint that nurse from healthy parents often easily nurse until 3 to 5 years of age, and in some cultures the weaning age is typically closer to 7 to 10 years. Just as infants nurse more than toddlers, the frequency of nursing tends to continue to decline with age. Many 3 to 5-year old's nurse every few days, rather than daily or multiple times per day like their 2 to 3-year-old counterparts.

Regardless of what others do, you should start considering now what sounds like an ideal time frame for you. You might just leave it open ended. Things most parents consider when thinking on this are often around teething, returning to work, returning to their "normal" non-lactating body, and spacing of future children. Sometimes the ideal time frame in your mind will center around the child's developmental phase or other personal reasons. The right choice is extremely personal, my hope is that you make it from an educated place.

Many parents often think that the burdens of breastfeeding are the same in infancy as toddlerhood, and this is incorrect. It is logistically less demanding to nurse a toddler than a newborn. There is less effort to maintain supply, pumping when separated is no longer needed. Toddlers nurse on average 2-5 times per day versus the 8-12 times per day of a newborn. I find these factors important to note as most people are uninformed on the differences.

Many people assume teething will create a huge barrier to breastfeeding success or think that it is an ideal time to wean. Teething is often feared because of the assumption of discomfort and biting, but this does not always happen. A good latch prevents teeth from being felt. Many babies do not even bite when teething, but they do nurse more frequently to seek comfort. Seeing as that teething can begin around 2-3 months, it may not be the wisest place to draw your line in the sand. I would suggest not assuming it will be a problem before there is an actual problem to address.

Returning to work might pose more of a challenge for some parents than others, depending on their work environment and personal feelings. Regardless of whether pumping at work can be made practical, a person may decide the hassle is just not worth it to them. It requires a lot of logistical challenges like hauling supplies, cleaning supplies, proper milk storage, leaking at work, and finding the time to pump. So, some parents stop nursing when they go back to work.

This decision can be influenced in shared custody arrangements, as well. If your former partner does not support breastfeeding or uses sabotaging breastfeeding to hurt you it will be harder to continue. There are usually ways to protect and preserve breastfeeding relationships, even when babies sometimes get bottles and formula without your expressed permission. It can be helpful in these cases to involve a professional third party to help come to agreements and make plans that make everyone happy. Sometimes the courts have to get involved, and not all judges rule wisely and fairly in favor of the child's best interests. If you have an abusive or narcissistic ex-partner or caregiver for your child, be prepared to face some difficulties with this.

Many parents are eager to stop nursing in order to have a non-pregnant and non-lactating body because of the physical demand and over-stimulation it can cause. Additionally, some parents want a break from lactation before their next pregnancy. It might be required for some females to stop lactation in order to ovulate, or to start fertility treatments.

Some parents think about how their child might be behaving developmentally around the age they want to wean. For example, one might decide they are comfortable nursing a 1 to 2-year-old because they might only nurse 3 to 5 times in 24 hours, and they can handle that demand. One also might decide that nursing a 2 to 3-year-old is still helpful for tantrums, as a parenting tool. Alternatively, one might find nursing past a certain age is just uncomfortable for them. There is much to consider when setting your goals.

Each facet of your life that is affected by nursing should be considered when setting your nursing goals. There should also be room left for the child and their decisions. You might plan to nurse through 3 years but have a child that weans at 2 years. You might plan to only nurse 6 months, but both enjoy it so much you go on to 1 year. Just remember the goals you make, for whatever reasons, are valid and worth pursuing. Also remember it is okay to change and adjust your goals. It might be necessary to adjust your goals if things unfold differently than you planned, and being open to that will help take away some of the sting and the shock of that reality when you are living it. Establishing a relationship with a lactation consultant can help you on your journey to meet whatever goals you have, but only you will be able to sit with yourself and ask yourself what you can live with and what is healthiest for you.

Decisions around how and what to feed your baby the first few months of their life is just the beginning of where you will start to experience the phenomenon known as "mom guilt." I feel like this is applicable to all parents. These feelings may even creep up during pregnancy and through labor and delivery. When you decide to breastfeed, you feel guilty for robbing others of the chance to bottle feed. When you bottle feed, you feel guilty for not breastfeeding. When you formula feed you might feel guilty for not pumping breastmilk. These examples are not true for every parent, but they represent the idea of the impossible dilemmas we are faced with because we have so much pressure on ourselves to do this perfectly, and the examples are endless.

Each decision you make as a parent for years to come will be muddled with (what is likely irrational) guilt. The feelings indicate you care, you are trying, you love your baby, and you are willing to take a hard look at yourself and see if there is room for improvement. This can lead down a slippery slope of self-doubt, though. It can help to write out logistical pros and cons, and pick either the least offensive choice or the one with the most benefits. Pick what you can live with. I always suggest picking the choices that you will be happy with 20 years from now. Placing a lens of an entire childhood over the small decisions can help you figure out which choices you feel the best about.

There is no doubt the pressure modern parents face to do things perfectly is immense. It seems no choice you make will be met without someone giving a contrary opinion of why you should have chosen differently. Guilt also surfaces when our internal feelings or behaviors do not match up with our expectations, especially for things like not instantly bonding with the baby. As with all trials, it is an opportunity to grow. Many parents find they really learn about themselves and go through intense personal growth in the early years of parenting.

Life in Relation to Breastfeeding

Costs of breastfeeding

Breastfeeding is not free—your time is money. Time is also used for bringing quality to our life. We spend our time with our friends, our partners, and our family. We spend our time taking care of our bodies and minds, exploring hobbies and interests. Breastfeeding being "free" is another patriarchal attitude that needs to be squashed. The message that parents should sacrifice their time to breastfeed because "it is free" also sends the message that a parent's time is value-less, and this message has been targeted at women for a long time. It implies that how they spend their time is completely irrelevant compared to the needs of their family and infant. I believe finding balance is possible, and even more possible in today's modern society versus the past. We are seeing attitudes shift in caretaker expectations, and we see an increase in the value we place on child-rearing as well as the invisible load of caretaking.

In today's world our time is the most valuable asset. If we look at the math, a newborn eating 30 minutes on each breast (1 hour), 8-12 times in 24 hours is about 8-12 hours for time spent just sitting and nursing. It is awfully hard to be somewhat forced to sit still, especially when you are accustomed to being able to do whatever you want or need relatively immediately. This can be really hard after the injuries to the vulva, as well. It will be physically and mentally challenging. This is a difficult sacrifice the first 4-6 weeks postpartum, because you are at the whim of an erratic on-demand feeding schedule. It makes it hard to plan errands, or self-care. This is especially hard for parents with high energy, high productivity, anxiety, attention deficit disorder, or post-traumatic stress disorder. Sure, you will eventually learn to multi-task a bit. You will be shamed for trying by some people; they expect you to just stare at your baby at every feeding session. This is actually fun for some sessions, to get to know their features and smell their sweet head. However, doing this 8-12 hours a day while sleep deprived is a bit unrealistic. I believe parents who might struggle with this should have flexibility built into their feeding plans to avoid unnecessary stress around the process.

Eventually, most babies do become more efficient at nursing, and their pattern more predictable. Usually, they will have gone from nursing 20 to 30 minutes on each breast down to 10 to 15. If you are super lucky and have a great flow and a very efficient nursling, it can be 5 to 10 minutes on each breast. This is when you will likely call your lactation consultant in a panic, worried that the baby is refusing your breast, or not eating enough.

One facet of losing time for other things is the time lost with friends and family. Often, many people find their family and friends come around a lot less often than they were expecting. When your spouse or partner returns to work it can also be a huge hit to how much social interaction you get. It is a common theme among new parents to feel lonely and isolated. Many parents find themselves more friendly and talkative in public with strangers, because they are craving connection. It is wired into the human species to crave and seek connection. It always has been, and always will be, critical to our survival.

Loneliness may not be exacerbated by nursing, but in some ways it can be. If you have family and friends who are not used to being around nurslings they may be very uncomfortable around you; or you might feel uncomfortable around them while nursing because of negative comments they make about it, or you might want to avoid them seeing your exposed mammae. Sometimes our cultural conditioning of avoiding letting another person see our breasts is a powerful reason that keeps us from socializing while breastfeeding. If you are facing multiple nursing challenges that can often become the main focus of your daily activities, and you might obsess and hyper-focus on breastfeeding and forget your need to connect. Additionally, regardless of how you feed most people will only ask about the baby, and not you. This can drive the isolated feelings further.

I do not believe we were meant to raise children in such isolation. To say "it takes a village" to raise a child is true, but we no longer live in villages. Our modern way of life has us very disconnected from each other, and child rearing has become a compartmentalized part of life—rather than the main focus of everyone's life. People used to have babies at a younger age on average and have many more babies in their lifetime then the modern parent. They were constantly nursing one baby then the next, all while regularly interacting with other people within their village, throughout the day. They had helping hands with their babies, and the chores. Now, many people often feel the need to hide away while nursing, and they miss many opportunities for connection. The sight of nursing infants has become less common, and less engrained as part of daily life while in public. Our bodies have evolved under the practices of collective caretaking, and parenting without a village goes against millions of years of evolution. Trying to raise children without a village is not a healthy or realistic expectation for the human species. It sets us up for being lonely, overwhelmed, and frustrated.

It has only been in very recent history that the breast was so hidden or hyper-sexualized, and it is not so in every culture. We have collectively moved towards considering it immodest to show the breast in many cultures. There is a current cultural shift back to normalizing and de-sexualizing the breast. Breastfeeding for most of our history had nothing to do with modesty or sex. It is only because the breast has become so hidden due to the popularity of formula feeding that we had temporarily and collectively shifted our view to it not being acceptable to nurse a baby in front of other people. The less we see the breast, the more shocking it seems to see it in daily life. There is an awareness and movement to normalize the image of a nursing baby on an exposed breast, because it is most logical to incorporate this frequent and necessary event back into our daily lives so that we can stop putting an undue burden on a nursing parent. This puts modern parents in the crossfire of the cultural shift. While you will encounter supportive people, you will still also encounter people who believe the breast should be hidden. It becomes another burden for a modern breastfeeding parent to be a part of the movement that normalizes breastfeeding in public again, as it puts them at risk for harassment.

The support of our immediate village is crucial to breastfeeding success. Sometimes our immediate family is not supportive of our goals. Most of us no longer cluster together with extended family the way we used to, so this is no longer how our support system is built. Most of us no longer have a sister close by to wet nurse our child so we can have a walk with our spouse or go run an errand. Our grandmothers and aunts are no longer just a holler away. They do not surround us and encourage us to expose our breast to feed our babies. They do not flock to us, several at a time, to help cook and clean and hold the baby so that we can bathe for a few minutes in peace. It is no wonder we have had an increase in postpartum mood disorders, and modern primary care-taking parents are more stressed than even a few decades ago.

A lot of this work is left up to the modern-day partner, who often knows little of caretaking or the demands on a freshly postpartum partner. There are partners that know how to take care of you and help, which is lovely but not yet the norm. A new parent should not have to worry about teaching their partner how to care for them while they are learning how to take care of themselves and take care of a child—but it is often the case. This is another topic best approached during or before pregnancy, rather than waiting to learn "on the job."

Some partners refuse to learn or to help, and the feeding parent is left carrying alone the burden of what was once completed by a village. Consider carefully when you have children, or more children, with someone if they can be a fair substitute for a village. There are some relationships broken by the weight of how hard this can be. It can be another unspoken cost.

Under this topic I also want to include a great cost that can present when older siblings are adjusting to a new sibling. The cost of time with them. This is a hard pill to swallow when you get into your second breastfeeding relationship because you have a routine and connection with your older child that is suddenly interrupted frequently throughout the day.

It is easy to incorporate all the children into a new routine with ease if you lead by example. Bring them with you to your "nursing spot" and let them sit with you and play or read a book together. Stash your nursing spot with snacks (for both of you), drinks, toys, books, and the remotes. Just show them attention in modified ways and keep them included. They can help with diaper changes and finding blankets and toys for baby. Do not feel bad if you send them to grandma's, daycare, or to the park with their other parent. Do not feel guilty for one second if they have more screen time than usual. Children are resilient and flexible; have faith in that. What you do for a few months to survive will go by in a blink, and then you will develop a new normal.

There is also a strange pull for many parents to make their breastfeeding experiences fair amongst each of their children. For example, if you only breastfeed your first 6 months, you might stop with your second at 6 months solely for fairness and not because you actually want to. Alternatively, many parents torture themselves to get to one year because they got there easily with their older child. If you find yourself facing these thoughts, I want you to know it is normal to have fear around this. It is also unlikely your children will care when they are adults, nor will they develop dramatically differently from each other. I have never heard children argue over who is loved most because they were nursed the longest. It is also not the only factor that influences their development. It is okay to give yourself permission to be open and flexible with each breastfeeding relationship and treat them individually from one another.

Self-care is another great cost that is lost with our time. If your baby spends an average amount of time eating that is about

8-12 hours less per day that you have available to devote to finding time for self-care. Multi-tasking and firmly setting boundaries are now top on your list of mastery. This can be challenging for people who are not used to having to firmly set boundaries in order to have their needs met. Taking time for self-care is one of the best ways to avoid caregiver burn-out, so contemplate how you will fit this into your new lifestyle before the baby comes. There is no need to martyr yourself to breastfeeding, or to parenting in general for that matter. Self-care does not have to be big grand gestures; it includes making sure you have enough food and water throughout the day. It can include making sure you get a 5-minute shower every day. It might include making sure you have your pain medications, your nipple balm, your peri-bottle, your perineal cool pads, and your tuck's pads always handy. Maybe for you it means painting your face and wearing your most stylish outfits, even if it is to just sit at home. It might mean making sure you get some time outside to get fresh air every day, to sit or to walk. Balance is possible, it takes a determined effort, planning, self-awareness, and setting clear boundaries. That includes cutting out any unnecessary extras that do not bring you health, be it mental or physical.

You will do well to remember, and remind your support people, that self-care that is needed for your physical, mental, and emotional well-being is not the same as getting a break. Getting an actual break from the invisible and visible load of parenthood should be a separate and distinct event from our small self-care rituals. Self-care should not be thought of as a luxury, but just what it sounds like, taking care of yourself. Self care means different things to different people, depending on their priorities, energy levels, and mental health. Having time and money for luxuries can benefit our mental health, but they would not be the only way to care for ourselves. Getting a real break is a form of self-care, but it is also letting people care *for* you because you will need the help of others in order to take a break.

Everyone should get breaks from their work. This includes working parents and stay at home parents, and other primary care-takers, too. So, taking a break from caretaking should not involve running errands, doing chores, basic hygiene, or doing any tasks that meet other people's needs. A real break means you are getting to do whatever it is you want to do that relaxes you and meets your needs. A break should not involve multi-tasking. Good examples of proper breaks might be 30 minutes of sitting alone in your house reading a book while your partner takes the rest of the family to the park, going to the spa and getting a treatment you do not normally get, grabbing coffee with a friend, going on a hike alone, going to a weekly painting class, or spending the night in a hotel alone to get some solid sleep.

Your partner needs breaks too, and you should both have equal opportunity to take them. You should both be getting time to have a hobby and do things that do not involve taking care of someone else's needs. If your partner is getting more break-time than you, you need to set boundaries around your break times and insist that you get them, too. Our hobbies and breaks should never be at the expense of exploiting our partners, and if that is happening it should be addressed.

The extreme physical, mental, and emotional challenges of parenting infants and toddlers often leave one or both part-ners feeling taken for granted, overlooked, taken advantage of, not loved, and burnt out. Most healthy partnerships would benefit from couples counseling during this transition, because, seriously, it is a doozy.

In addition to the time lost to self-care, you might lose chances of being cared for. When you would normally go to your mother's every Saturday to be cooked dinner, maybe now you are staying home with the baby for a few months and not con-tinuing this habit. While your partner would normally rub your feet every night while you watched a show together, you are now spending your evening consoling a fussy baby during the witching hour. Many examples of this can creep in and caring for your baby will take over all your old habits that gave you time to be shown love through action and physical touch or affection.

You might need to talk to the people who take care of you and remind them that you still need these things. Ask your mom to bring over the dinner. Ask your partner to rub your feet while you nurse the baby. Ask for affection. Ask for food. Ask for help. Do not let your needs be forgotten or overlooked in the fog of the newborn storm. You care for the baby. The village will care for you.

Another lifestyle change and cost will revolve around how hungry and thirsty you are compared to normal. Your body is expending more energy than usual in order to create milk. When you have the hormonal boost that lets your milk flow you will also experience a surge in hunger and thirst. This is your reminder to take care of yourself. It can help you to have a drink and snack basket set up next to where you will typically sit to nurse. Generally, lactating people need about 500 more calories per day than normal. It helps to curb severe hunger pangs if those calories are more protein and fat than carbs and sugar.

I mentioned before that your baby might not take a bottle or have a bottle strike. This is a "cost" of breastfeeding when you do not introduce it as an option for your infant early enough in their development nor keep it a part of their routine. It can cost you peace of mind, flexibility with care-taking options, and being able to run errands, go on trips, or work outside of the home. If you anticipate any separation from your baby this is a skill you want them to have. This includes being separated for date nights. Introducing a bottle by 4 to 6 weeks and then continuing to give a bottle a few times a week can help prevent this. It is much harder to convince a 6 month old baby who has not had a bottle since they were 2 weeks old that this is an acceptable way to eat versus an infant who has routinely taken bottles since 4 weeks of age.

The time you spend obsessing about baby's intake is also a "cost" factor. What is this costing your emotional health? Are you someone who worries and obsesses in general? For many parents being able to see and calculate intake can be calming to their fears. These parents usually end up exclusively bottle feeding in order to achieve that close monitoring. That is something I might encourage a parent to explore with their therapist, as we have not closely calculated infants' intake for thousands of years —this is a very recent and possibly counter-productive practice. It should be enough information to count the daily diaper output and weigh the baby weekly. Trust should be placed in the infant's ability to cue for its needs and follow its' instincts. There is no shame if you cannot emotionally handle the unknown and need to bottle feed to feel safe and secure, I would just implore you to explore why you think you need that.

It is beneficial in the early days if there are risk factors to closely monitor intake with more scrutiny in order to ensure a baby survives and thrives. This often includes waking the baby to feed and encouraging the baby to eat every 2 hours on schedule, and more often if they cue to feed more frequently. After things are stable it is less important to monitor intake so closely. Once the baby is gaining well, alert enough to wake to feed on their own body's cues, and well hydrated they can be trusted to be followed for their intrinsic feeding and satiety cues. This means you will no longer have to wake them to eat, and you can follow the feeding pattern that they instinctively cue for. This is often when the baby is a few weeks old and the milk supply is more established. The babies typically do not regress once they are stable and progressing well with feeding. This can be a hard transition to switch from scrutiny to trust, and I am not suggesting it is abnormal for that change to be hard. You can wait until you get the all-clear from your IBCLC and pediatrician, to make sure you do not make this change too soon. We can generally trust baby's instincts and for them to let us know in behavior and diaper count if their intake is adequate or not. Learning what is normal can be calming enough to those anxieties, without making the breastfeeding relationship harder than it needs to be.

Weight gain and other hormonal and physical changes

There are lucky people that lose weight while breastfeeding. I am sure you have heard about the myth of a slimmer figure being touted as one of the top reasons to breastfeed. However, the biological design is that females should store fat in case of famine in order to continue to breastfeed and help their offspring survive. Many lactating people find that they have a more challenging time shedding extra stored fat that they do not want, or they find it altogether impossible. The idea that we need to be slender while pregnant and breastfeeding goes entirely against our body's encoded instructions for survival of our offspring.

Most nursing parents experience extreme hunger and postpartum nursing cravings, similar to pregnancy cravings and surges in hunger. This is because our hormones are encouraging us to feast, if the food is available. Being able to store fat on our body has a survival benefit because if we experience a famine, our body will still be able to produce plenty of milk from our fat stores to ensure our offspring's survival for longer, at least until an alternative food source can be found.

On the other hand, many women find their hormones cause them to lose weight rapidly and they are unable to keep up with eating enough calories to continue nursing. Often they are spending an inordinate amount of time trying to eat, and still not keeping on weight. If your weight becomes dangerously low, or you develop certain health risks, you might have to wean prematurely or reduce how much you breastfeed.

You will either lose weight, gain weight, or have a stable weight. There is no way to predict what your genetic encoding favors during pregnancy and while nursing until you are in the thick of it. Forget the social constructs around excess body fat that require a separate book to discuss, and just think for yourself if this will bother you or not. You will have to weigh the temporary risk of excess weight gain (or being unable to shed weight) versus the lifelong benefits to you and the baby. This can be a serious struggle for some parents, and you should not feel ashamed if it is too great a cost for you.

Many postpartum parents are targeted by people trying to help you lose weight and get your pre-baby body back. Your body will never be the same, even if you are thin. There are a lot of useless and even dangerous products that try to override your genetic code to hold onto fat when in your child-bearing years. Finding a healthy way to eat and exercise during pregnancy and postpartum will be helpful, but you may need to adjust your expectations and learn to love this temporary new body. If not after pregnancy, after weaning you will return to a hormonal state that makes it easier to lose unwanted extra body fat if that is your goal. Many people are surprised to find they do not even mind the curvier figure that comes with child-bearing.

Exercising is likely to cross your mind when thinking of health and fitness goals; and it is generally safe once you are cleared by your obstetrician or midwife about 4-8 weeks postpartum. Being cleared will depend on how much you exercised while pregnant, how you labored and delivered, and how quickly you are recovering. It is unlikely to reduce your milk supply if you exercise in moderation and make sure to adequately hydrate and eat enough nutritional food.

Other than carrying around more body fat than before, your body's appearance can change many other ways. Your skin may stretch so far that you develop stretch marks, your hormones might cause your feet to grow in size, a dark line might appear on your belly, a dark mark might appear on your face, you might see a change in the shape of your hips, your stomach muscles may be more round than flat, your skin might be more oily or acne prone, your skin might be more dry, and your hair color and texture may change too. It can be overwhelming and shocking to see the new you. It is okay to struggle with these changes or not like them, and it is okay to embrace them and enjoy them. There is no right way to respond, but I do encourage you to practice gratitude to ease the discomfort around the changes. When we focus on thanking our body for all that it does, it makes it harder to focus on all that it is not.

Some other hormonal changes include the lack of estrogen causing decreased libido and vaginal dryness. These are not symptoms that exist in isolation but are likely to play a part in your sexually intimate relationship. It is important to be prepared for this change and have open dialogue with your partner about expecting these changes and how it is not a reflection of your love or attraction for them. You might even experience finding your partner's natural smell off-putting during pregnancy and nursing. This is likely because your body is trying to protect you and your baby by avoiding too close of subsequent pregnancies.

Nursing also can cause delay of ovulation and your cycles; this can compound the issue of decreased libido as ovulation is typically accompanied by a libido surge. The cycle is often irregular when it does return, and often does not return for many months. For some people it does not return until weaning is complete. Breastfeeding can also be negatively affected by the hormonal cycling such that there is a supply dip right before or during your period, a change in taste of your milk, and nipple tenderness. These are usually temporary and return to normal after a few days. Usually calcium and magnesium supplements help counter this dip.

Those who are susceptible to having hormones influence their acne, headache pattern, eczema, auto-immune conditions, or other illnesses might find that nursing either exacerbates or suppresses these conditions. Sometimes the hormonal changes even cause people to develop new food allergies or a different hair texture and pattern. It can be different with each person and what might trigger these conditions or changes within them and can vary with each pregnancy they have.

It is important to know also that the continuation of some pregnancy discomforts like not getting to sleep on your stomach, aching or stiff joints, or auto-immune flares might continue through the nursing relationship for some people. If you look forward to sleeping on your stomach again, that might not be possible because it makes you more prone to clogs if you compress the breast tissue by sleeping in that position, and it might make you leak all over the bed. For joint pains, it is especially prevalent for postpartum females to have aching wrists and there is a condition of postpartum carpal tunnel syndrome symptoms or arthritis, or "mother's thumb," "de Quervain's tenosynovitis" and it is from hormones and repetitive mechanical motions. Treatment is rest, ice, compression, elevation, non-steroidal anti-inflammatory medications, stretching, splinting, and maybe occupational or physical therapy and massage. Occupational or physical therapy can teach you to strengthen muscles around the joints to provide more stability to them and reduce some of the pain. If it is general pain to all of your joints the treatment is the same, and it's also from the hormonal and chemical changes of pregnancy. Some of the pain can linger or get worse while you are nursing. Some of the hormonal change helps your joints shift and relaxes your ligaments for the changes of carrying the baby, and then opening the hips for labor, and it helps with being more flexible for odd nursing positions. Sometimes the pain is from weight gain, too. It serves some biological purposes, and it is usually generalized to all the joints, but sometimes the pain can be more focused in certain joints like the hands, wrists, or hips.

For some people joint pain is a flare of an autoimmune disorder like arthritis, that the hormones make worse. Females are more susceptible to autoimmune conditions due to our hormones, and especially when they fluctuate like with pregnancy and lactation. Some people develop autoimmune conditions during big hormonal changes. For example, many postpartum parents develop arthritis, thyroiditis, and lupus. If the joints are red and hot, it might be autoimmune. Seeing your healthcare provider for labs and assessments can help you rule out autoimmune conditions or underlying injuries and get a treatment plan. Sometimes these issues resolve after weaning but sometimes they remain a chronic problem. Treatment for chronic conditions might be more complicated like with additional medications or trigger point injections, on top of the other suggestions. Some joint aches, depending on the cause, feel better with heat therapy versus cold therapy, and your provider can suggest medications specific to your problem, so getting a personalized plan is helpful.

Another physical discomfort many nursing parents notice is neck, shoulder, and back pain. This can be due to poor body mechanics, not having ergonomic positioning, having your head hung forward many hours of the day, sitting frequently, and muscles being challenged differently. It is also due to your spine and abdomen being held in a completely different pattern and position when you are carrying a baby versus when you are not. The core is weakened from the pregnancy and the delivery, and it can feel odd and even painful to try to stand upright. It is important to set up nursing so that you are sitting upright with square shoulders, and bringing baby to you rather than slouching to bring your breast to the baby, or you will make these neck and shoulder pains worse. You also want proper support under the baby so that you are not holding all of the weight of their body. Eight pounds does not seem heavy, until you hold it for 30 minutes straight. Stretching out the neck, hips, abdomen, and low back daily will also help.

The relaxin hormone that surges in pregnancy leads to these musculoskeletal changes like ligament relaxation which helps our hips open for labor. It lingers while we are nursing, which is likely to help our bodies be more flexible. It can allow our tailbone to shift out of the baby's way as they descend down the birth canal, which leaves that joint sore as well. Most people have very sore hips, pelvic bones, and tail bones after delivery. It is more so if you deliver vaginally, but still happens when you deliver via cesarean. The muscle strain and hormonal changes also contribute to some pelvic floor weakness which can cause some urine incontinence to linger, and cause gas to pass without warning. This is especially true when you sneeze or cough. It is especially bad when your pelvic floor is in shock the first few days postpartum, and you may just release a bladder full of urine without realizing it. It also lends to having some uterine pro-lapse, which should ideally heal and firm up after a few months. However, if you are still having these issues several months postpartum it will be time to discuss pelvic floor physical ther-apy or surgical correction with your provider.

When there is hormonal fluctuation there is also some-times hot flashes! Many breastfeeding parents often say they are very warm, and it is not just due to the body heat of the baby that is on their chest, the heat from metabolism increase, or heat from within the mammae. Many postpartum females have night sweats the first few weeks as hormones adjust, and the hot flashes might last the entire nursing journey.

Another thing that surprises many postpartum females is quite a bit of hair loss around 3 to 6 months postpartum. This will happen if you breastfeed or not. It may happen again when you wean! This is because of your hormones! Some people lose so much hair that they have some bald-spots, and if this is hap-pening you need to have your primary care doctor check your thyroid function, as postpartum females are at high risk for thyroid dysfunction. With each pregnancy and nursing relation-ship the texture and color of your hair may change. You will be surprised what little (and big) things you notice are influenced by hormones.

The hormonal changes of nursing also influence how you smell, how your bodily fluids smell, your sense of smell, how much you sweat, how hot you feel, the texture of your skin, your mood, your periods, and many other things. Many things are similar to pregnancy, especially in the fourth trimester. Most of these changes continue to benefit the survival and connection of the parent-infant dyad. Some of these changes do not seem to serve a purpose, like continuing to feel phantom kicks in your belly and being more susceptible to hemorrhoids.

Females experiencing a stronger sense of smell is likely to the benefit of being able to detect spoiled food more easily, just like in pregnancy. Most new female parents also have more sensitive hearing and sleep very lightly. This likely is to the benefit of attending to the baby's needs more readily as well as detecting environmental threats more easily. Your still round and swollen belly after delivery makes the perfect resting place for the newborn at the breast, and for some people it can be harder to reduce their belly until after they wean. Everything that pregnancy and nursing changes can change again after weaning, but some things are permanent! There really is no pattern to what changes persist, you will just have to wait and see as it changes from person to person, and with each pregnancy.

During weaning, people often experience dramatic changes. Common experiences are weaning depression, hair loss, hormonal acne, hot flashes, breast pain, and many other uncomfortable symptoms. Weaning depression is just like other depressions. Emotional and hormonal changes make the process of weaning hard, even if done gradually. Many people experience physical discomfort as well as sadness, an urge to cry, loss of enjoyment of foods and hobbies, difficulty sleeping or wanting to sleep more than usual, feeling unmotivated, and lacking the energy or motivation to maintain usual hygiene habits. The emotional and hormonal changes can also induce anger, rage, intrusive thoughts, or a resurgence of mood disorders or physical disease that was being alleviated during breastfeeding. For example, if nursing was calming your arthritis you may have horrible flares while weaning. This is not normalized or discussed often enough and is a very real and expected experience when weaning.

Breastfeeding and Pumping Paraphernalia

There is an exceedingly long list of all the things you could buy in the world that claim to help make breastfeeding and pumping easier. There are supplements, breast warmers, clog busters, pumping bras, special flanges, reusable milk storage bags, leaking milk catchers, and many more paraphernalia. While some of them can surely be helpful, you may also have household items that serve as a perfect substitute. Breastfeeding does not have to be ruined by financial barriers; you can get creative.

Examples might be a breast warmer that can be re-created by microwaving some rice that you wrap up into a sock, or a vibration tool to break up a clog could be replaced by a personal massager. For some people, the luxury of warming breast massagers is very helpful as it combines the effects of warmth and massage, and is in a convenient shape. This might be preferred for a person who is not responding well to pumping, is using a wearable pump that makes massaging awkward, or has implants or another need for extra stimulation. It is easy to fall prey to the clever marketing and think we need every little thing, and what you will want or need will depend on your personal preferences and goals. It is a good idea to ask your lactation consultant or friends what is helpful, what can be replaced with household items, and maybe even what they are ready to hand-off that they no longer have use for. These are the perfect kinds of questions to ask in a peer group, on social media, or in a chat platform!

Most end up using nipple cream, balm, or butter. It is important to know that if you have sensitivity to wool you will also likely be sensitive to lanolin containing products, because it is made from the oil off of a sheep's teat. I see many patients slather on lanolin for months with unexplained nipple tenderness. For the most part with these nipple products you need trial and error of which works best for you. Ingredients like coconut oil have antifungal and antibacterial properties. The main reason these products work though is because they keep the microscopic cracks in the nipple moist and provide a barrier so that the nipple skin can heal with less friction from your bra or pads. When a nipple injury is present, like scabbing and cracks, hydrogel pads are superior to the creams for healing. You may need prescription nipple cream if the damage is severe enough.

Having a proper fitting flange is likely more important than having a flange with a special feature or material, but studies have not been done on the newer soft silicone flanges versus the older harder ones. It is best to wait until after delivery, and again a few days after, and again a few weeks postpartum to measure your nipples to determine flange size. This is due to the effect of estrogen on nipple size. When you are pregnant the high estrogen makes the nipples larger and darker. In the postpartum period it is normal for them to shrink and change in elasticity. Proper flange fit should not be guessed or estimated, as it is critical to avoiding injury and optimizing output. A flange that is too large will pull too much areola into the tunnel, which will kink off duct flow and can reduce supply and lead to clogging. A flange that is too small will not only block some flow but also cause blisters from friction.

Choosing the pump itself can be overwhelming as more pumps hit the market yearly. Consumer reviews can be immensely helpful in this process. If your insurance only covers a few specific brands and models, that can help narrow things down. You also can pay out of pocket if you have a specific one in mind. Ideally your pump will be able to toggle in and out of several modes, speeds, and suction levels. Even better if it does it automatically and is very highly customizable. Deciding to buy one of the most convenient and newest style of pumps that allow you to move about freely while pumping can take one of the greatest frustrations of pumping away. Unfortunately, not all insurance companies cover pumps equally and there may be a financial block to access here, as these pumps are considered a luxury and not the standard. Pumps are not usually something you want to buy used, but if you must then choose what is called a "closed system" pump. There are also hospital grade double electric pumps that are shown to be superior in studies when establishing milk supply in the early postpartum days. These are often too expensive for most people to purchase but they are able to be shared, leading to the common practice of them being available for rent temporarily. My best advice for choosing a pump would be first to explore the options of what is covered by your insurance, and second thoroughly read through as many consumer reviews and comparisons as you can find. Often choosing the best pump feels overwhelming due to so many options. This is something I would suggest investigating while pregnant.

Bras are something most females wear, and they usually feel bras are a need when nursing and pumping. There are pumping bras, nursing bras, and combination bras. Some people just stick to regular bras and pull them out of the way. Some just use tank tops and make it work. The girls appreciate the extra support when they are heavier and fuller, and when pumping it is pretty important to get a pumping bra, or make one, due to hands-on pumping being so much more effective. Hands-on pumping is simply compressing and massaging the mammae while pumping.

Thus, pumping bras can be greatly beneficial when you need the flange held to the breast so that you can actually use your hands to enhance pumping, rather than using them to hold the flanges. Hands-on pumping is a studied and proven way to increase milk production. A pumping bra can be created by simply cutting holes in an old sports bra, to stick the flanges through. Though perhaps not as practical for when you return to work, it can be a perfect solution for a parent pumping at home.

Nursing clothes, nursing bras, and pumping bras are another expense that you may or may not incur, but you will definitely start to dress with consideration to how easily you can access your mammae. Nursing clothes are not a must-have, but they do make life a little easier. You may be happy to use the two-shirt method, or just pull your regular clothes out of the way. Typically following pregnancy and during lactation, a larger bra is needed, so if you wear one you may not be able to escape that expense.

Other choices around pumping paraphernalia might include how many pieces you actually need, and paraphernalia used to clean and sterilize. It is likely that no one will mention to you that you need to replace the valves and membranes in the pump parts frequently, as they wear out with use, and this can affect your pump output if not done at regular intervals. How often will depend on how often you pump. When you are pumping several times per day it can be helpful to have several sets to cut down on needing to wash everything between each pump session. Although not CDC approved, many parents will pump and then store their flange pieces in the refrigerator between pump sessions after putting the pumped milk into a separate container. If you have a preemie or immunocompromised baby this "fridge hack" can be riskier. The thought process behind the fridge hack is that milk can be good in the fridge for 5 days, so 24 hours of pulling the parts in and out of the fridge should inhibit bacterial growth enough to be safe, especially as fresh milk with fresh antibodies is pumped into the parts at each session. Decisions like that will be at your discretion. There are also, however, cleaning wipes and sprays that can work in a pinch between pump sessions. If you find yourself needing to sterilize you can use sterilizing machines, the dishwasher with a parts basket, microwavable sterilizing bags and microwavable plastic kits that utilize steam. It is important to note that not all pump manufacturers approve the microwavable methods, as it can warp parts. There are also cold sterilization tablets that avoid the use of heat. It is also important to note that you only need to sterilize parts the first time you use them, and not daily or with each use, unless pumping for a preemie or immunocompromised baby. Sterilizing may come into the picture again if you and baby are treated for thrush, because then you have to sterilize at each point of contact everything that touches your nipples or the baby's mouth. This would include pump parts, bottles, nipples, nipple shields, pacifiers, baby teething toys, baby spoons, and the like.

Speaking of nipple shields, they are another nursing tool that can be extremely helpful, but also very cumbersome. In the beginning they can help a weaker or tongue-tied baby get the latch they need in order to pull milk more efficiently. They can also act as a buffer for a painful latch, often reducing the pain felt in the nipples and reducing the damage to the nipples when the baby is injuring the nipples. They can also provide the firmer stimulation needed on the roof of the mouth to stimulate the suckle reflex for a baby reluctant to take a softer, smaller, shorter, or flatter nipple. They can become quite the hassle as they are tricky to get to stay put and you have to keep track of it and wash it after every use. You will come across lactation consultants who give them out like candy, and others who avoid them like the plague. However, I am of the mind that it is a tool to help you so if it is helpful to you—use it! There are no longer strict guidelines suggesting shields potentially being harmful because we no longer use the thick shields that diminished nipple stimulation in the past. Old studies that show this are just that, old and outdated. The thinner more flexible shields now often do not diminish stimulation and often help baby transfer more than they would without it. It is beneficial when you are using one to continually and frequently reassess if your baby is capable of latching and transferring without it. Often babies will decide on their own that the shield is just in the way and desire to nurse without it. This is often when they are a few months old and thus developmentally able to make the connection with the breast being where they latch and feed. They no longer require the stimulation of the suckling reflex in order to start the feed. If someone is suggesting the use of the shield, be sure to ask what it is helping with and how they plan to wean you off of it. Do not be afraid to use it temporarily, as for most babies it is possible to wean off its use eventually. If it is the difference between nursing with a shield or pumping, then I would opt to use the shield. If you are finding you need a shield, or having difficulty weaning from the shield, seek out an IBCLC to assess the latch or give you tips to wean off of it.

Other paraphernalia that might be promoted are baby scales. Parents might want to purchase one if they might wish to monitor weight gain without frequent outings to the clinic. Unfortunately, this is not always really needed, and marketing takes advantage of the fact that parents can become quite obsessed with weight gain. Retail infant scales are not sensitive enough at the typical consumer level to tell you exactly how much milk the baby is transferring, especially not in milliliters. Scales that go down to the grams or milliliters typically cost thousands of dollars and are sometimes available to rent. A more reasonable retail grade scale might do well to help you track weekly weight gain. It should be able to measure down to 0.25 to 0.5 ounces, which might be able to help with weighted feeds if you are feeding several ounces per feed. A scale meant to measure adult weight will not be sensitive enough for babies, as you are looking for weight differences in ounces, and adult scales are often off by pounds. There are 16 ounces per pound for reference, so that is a lot of room for error.

Many people will also try to sell you essential oils claiming they help with breastfeeding or common parenting woes. People that sell it will assure you it is safe for infants due to its high quality. Certified aromatherapists, essential oil therapists, and many healthcare providers warn against putting oils on infants—even if diluted. Certain oils like lavender and eucalyptus are thought to be dangerous. Lavender can be an endocrine disrupter and is a powerful medicinal herb even before being concentrated in an essential oil form. Eucalyptus and similar oils have been shown to negatively influence breathing regulation in infants and toddlers. The essential oils fennel and basil are also often sold to boost supply, and while they work temporarily it is not without a cost. The estrogenic effect of the fennel, especially combined with the lactation hormones, can increase your risk of breast cancer. Essential oils are powerful and useful tools and clearly illicit responses in on our bodies. Their being natural products does not automatically mean they are safe. As with dried herbal remedies, they can be dangerous, as are the essential oils of herbs. They should be used with extreme caution and your source of information on dosing and form of use should be someone certified in herbal or aromatic medicine, not just someone who is hoping you will buy their products. While they can be well-meaning, convincing, and speak with conviction, they are often caught giving unsafe advice.

When you continue nursing past the newborn stage you will face different challenges with nursing throughout the baby's developmental phases. Most parents find that after the first 2-3 months nursing actually becomes significantly easier. The steep learning curve starts to flatten, and the needs of the baby become slightly less demanding. In fact, no matter how you feed your baby, coming out of the fog of the fourth trimester feels like a different life has started. The first three months go by so slow when you are in the fog of the day in and day out, but at the same time they go by in a flash.

Babies often get more efficient at nursing as the months go by and take a shorter amount of time which always ends up worrying parents that their baby is not getting enough. When your supply down-regulates more closely to baby's demand around 12 weeks, this is also a common time for parents to worry about adequate milk supply. The baby will go through many growth spurts that have them nursing frequently for days, and this will also likely make you question your supply. Additionally, their rate of growth begins to slow so the amount of expected weight gain decreases and when this change occurs it can be alarming if you are not prepared for it.

Other than worries about sufficient supply you might get frustrated when normal baby behaviors influence how peaceful the nursing session is. The older baby gets distracted easily; looks away while still latched or pops on and off the breast to look around. When they pop off mid let-down this can create a large mess, as the milk will spray out onto the baby and your clothes. This behavior becomes more frequent around the time when parents are spending more time nursing out in public because they are eager to get out and about and not be at home so much. This can be a source of anxiety for some parents, especially when it feels like you are just getting comfortable with the idea of nursing in public.

Nursing in public is its own stressor because you will need to figure out for yourself what level of comfort you have with exposing your breast in public. It can be hard with cultural conditioning to tap into your instinct to respond to and feed your child, anywhere, at any time. This comes into play as soon as the baby is born, and you have to choose if you want visitors in the hospital or not. If you are uneasy about exposing your breasts when others are present, having visitors will interfere with allowing you to feed the baby on demand.

This is true when you are at home, too. You will have to make hard decisions to protect your safe space so that you can freely feed on demand without stress, and sometimes that means prohibiting visitors. Even if you have helpful and attentive visitors, which most people do not get, you might struggle with feeling like you have to play host when other people are in your house. If you cannot stop yourself from trying to clean your house, cook for guests, and be a generally dutiful host then you do not have to let people come over! Knowing your strengths and weaknesses and admitting to them can only help you as you move into this new phase of adulthood. If you fail to become self-aware and set the boundaries that you need it will jeopardize your mental and physical health, and likely sabotage breastfeeding success. Now, if it takes actually having people over to realize how much space you need, it is ok to change your mind and stop the visiting parade for a few days. It is okay to tell someone you love to stop coming over because it is stressing you out, for any reason. It is also okay to keep allowing visits if you find that you are getting a lot of help, rest, and comfort from the social interactions.

There are many options if you are not comfortable nursing in front of others but do want company. You can try using nursing covers, the two-shirt method, and nursing clothing. Of course, if you are comfortable, you can also just pull your breast out of your shirt without any extra steps or options. This decision process can also cause fights between partners when you have different ideas about what is appropriate. Your ideas and plans might change as you get more comfortable, or more insecure, and might change with each baby. Only you will be able to decide what you are comfortable with. Remember, you are the boss of your body; no one else.

After that first distracted phase in the first few months, you are introducing solids around 6 months, and balancing the food intake with protecting your milk supply. Sometimes the solid remnants in the mouth can be irritating to the skin on the nipples. It can become harder to distinguish what your child wants, now with more options available. They may not only want solids rather than breast, but their fussing might be because they are bored and want to play!

As you get to the stage of nursing an older baby, and especially nursing past a year, you will likely want to start teaching what are called "nursing manners." Just like you are slowly teaching table manners, you will teach your baby to respect your body and your boundaries around nursing. This might include teaching them to sign "milk" to indicate they want to nurse, rather than them tugging on your shirt. It might also include making rules, such as, "no milk until bedtime or naptime" if you are trying to limit nursing sessions.

You will likely start to face criticism or suggestions to wean, even as early as a few months postpartum, but especially the older your child gets. Nursing into toddlerhood is the biological norm, but not currently the societal norm in most cultures. It may shock you to even find healthcare professionals encouraging weaning before the biological norm, because we have strayed so far from nature in the past century, especially in healthcare.

There are always the odd suggestions to start replacing your human milk for your human child with cow milk or an alternative milk, made for another species. This is not only not necessary, but the practice was only started about 10,000 years ago so our bodies are not perfectly adapted to trying another species' milk. We also use to only do this when nutrition and hydration options were scarce. If you have breastmilk, there is no need to do this. Toddlers who have access to clean water, and a nutritious and plentiful diet get everything they need from nursing 2-3 times per 24 hours. If they are not nursing, they can add healthy fats and vegetable sources of calcium into their diet to replace the milk, and still do not need cow milk.

Traveling

Traveling while breastfeeding or providing breastmilk can be very logistically challenging. You might be going for pleasure or for work, so the challenges might not be the same for each circumstance. I will briefly mention some helpful tips.

When you drive, you will have to pull over to change and feed baby as driving while nursing can be fatal to you and baby if you crash. If you have a pump or pumped milk you will need a converter to allow you to plug in your pump or charge it, and a cooler to keep milk at the right temperature. Pumped bottles also cannot be safely fed while the car is in motion because the baby cannot be taken fast enough out of the seat if they start choking, and the bottle can become a projectile. Plan for the trip to take longer than usual or expected, because babies will need to be taken out of their seat frequently. It can be helpful to try to get in long stretches of driving when baby has their longest stretch of sleep, and take turns driving and sleeping with your travel companion.

For flying, it is helpful to feed baby during takeoff and descent to help equalize pressure in their ears. If you are pumping, be sure to pack extra pump parts and a mini cooler. The breast pump is considered medical equipment and does not count as your carry on. You might need to point this out to staff at the airport. Your liquid breastmilk is not subject to the 3 oz limit, but you will go through the line faster if it is frozen. Fresh milk has to be screened; frozen milk is usually just passed through. Baby wearing also helps keep baby calm and makes nursing more accessible.

Then, when you arrive at your destination you will be in a different space trying to re-create what happens at home, and this can be unsettling for parents and babies. Try to bring familiar items like blankets that smell like home, and noise machines or fans you usually have running. Have a plan for handling family or friends and how you will allow them to interact with your baby, and what you will do at feeding times.

Breastfeeding while working

Most postpartum females in countries without paid and protected maternity leave need to work outside of the home while also meeting their breastfeeding goals, which necessitates pumping or expressing milk when away from the baby. If you are not going to be working while still breastfeeding this section might not apply to you. Most parents choose pumping rather than hand expressing, to make it easier. Working parents need to get a bit of milk stashed away before returning to work and need to make sure the baby will take a bottle. Unfortunately, many women do not have political, legal, or cultural support that helps protect the nursing dyad. Without paid maternity leave like many other countries, breastfeeding rates suffer and drop off more quickly than the recommended 1-2 years (or longer) of nursing. The burden to keep the relationship going is on the lactating person, and is often not made easy due to social and cultural resistance as well as lack of legal protections. Decisions around breastfeeding might have the potential to impact your family financially.

Knowing if your baby will take a bottle or not is a common fear for parents who will be working outside of their home within the infant's first year of life. This is a common fear even if you do not have to go back to work, as you will likely want to know in the event of needing to leave the baby that they can be fed. Reasons might be emergent or practical, such as needing to go to an appointment where the baby cannot go with you. I think the best way to handle this is be proactive, introduce bottles early and often. I know, shocking from an IBCLC but it is true.

I wish I could tell the parents who come to me at 3 to 6 months to go back in time and stay on top of those bottle skills. Introducing 1 or 2 pump sessions and 1 or 2 bottles in the early weeks postpartum allow parents to get familiar with the pump, start building a freezer stash, ensure the baby will take a bottle, and get rest and breaks from time to time. I believe avoiding pumps and bottles for the first 6 weeks can be counter-productive to many modern parent's desires. Whether or not a lactation consultant wants you to avoid bottles and pumping is, to me, irrelevant. What matters is what the parents want, and what their long-term goals are. I rarely see these steps taken in moderation and under guidance to sabotage the establishment of breastfeeding. In fact, I find the rest that is facilitated for the feeding parent makes them more likely to continue to breastfeed than if they were exhausted and worn down without ever being given a chance to get a break or have a stretch of sleep longer than 2-3 hours for weeks on end.

The biological norm is to breastfeed, and an older baby is perfectly happy to do so when it is all they know. There is absolutely nothing wrong with keeping with this biological norm. However, when you need to return to work when they are 3-6 months old, they will not understand the desire to introduce the bottle, nor see the need. Most consultants will have some helpful tricks for you to get the baby to take a bottle, but do yourself a favor and let them have one early and often if you know they will likely ever need one in the first 6 months of life. The flexibility of feeding method is a great stress reducer for most parents. If we miss our opportunity or baby loses the bottle-feeding skill, then after 6 months we can move on to sippy cups, straw cups, and lots of solids when a parent has to be away. Many infants "reverse cycle" and will nurse more frequently when the parent is home to make up for the lost time apart.

When you are pumping because you are working it can be harder to maintain supply. One thing that helps is returning to work slowly, if possible. Return part time initially and ramp up your hours slowly over several weeks or several months. Ask if you can work part-time from home, if your type of work allows it.

When you are pumping more than nursing, you will see supply regulation, perceived as supply dips, at 3, 6, 9 and 12 months. As a pumping parent this will be more obvious, as the pumping output will decrease. Pumping both mammae at the same time, or double pumping, helps you have a stronger hormonal response and get more milk out. Power pumping every few days will help keep it boosted, as this mimics cluster feeding. Power pumping can be done several ways, but the idea is to have a few pump sessions very close together, about 10-50 minutes apart, rather than 2-3 hours apart like routine pumping or feeding.

The timing of supply regulation also often coincides with needing to reduce flange size. The further postpartum you are, the more your nipples will shrink. Fit is important to maximizing breast drainage. You will want the flange to fit your nipple and have some clearance around it, but not pull too much areola in. If you are uncertain of fit, see your lactation consultant for help with sizing.

There is also the emotional challenge around leaving your baby for many hours a day and fearing they will prefer their caretaker over you. While this is unlikely, it is a common fear many parents consider when thinking about going back to work.

Even if it is good for you financially and emotionally to work, it is still deeply engrained in our biology to want to be near our infants. So, fighting that, even when we know it is the best choice for us, is tricky. You might feel guilty if you are excited to go back to work, and this might be stemming from those strong biological drives as well as cultural conditioning.

Then there are the challenges once you actually get to work, even if you work from home. Some people, regardless of lawful protection, give females a hard time about pump breaks during work hours. Some co-workers of lactating parents have been found guilty of tossing or drinking breastmilk. The space the company provides might be unsanitary, not have a lock, or people will ignore the lock or privacy sign and interrupt you. This can be really hard for people who seek to avoid confrontation. Some employers and coworkers are not familiar with pumping protection laws, or they are, and they do not care. Sometimes the boss supports you, but coworkers are resentful because of your extra "breaks." They will not recognize the sacrifice or inconvenience. People can be very forward and rude in expressing their disapproval of pumping or breastfeeding, and they might do rude things like call it gross, or complain about you or your milk. It is disturbingly common, even when working with other lactating or formerly lactating people, to meet resistance and discouragement in the workplace. Sometimes our societal conditioning keeps us from even asking what we have a right to. It often puts parents in an unfair position of choosing to continue to work or choosing to continue to breastfeed. This is a conversation best approached before maternity leave. Be prepared to have to stand your ground but hope for wiser minds to prevail.

Your legal right is to have your employer provide a clean and private place to pump that has a lockable door and is not a bathroom. They are legally required to give you breaks, but not to pay you for them, as often and as long as you need. They are not exempt from this until they prove undue burden or file for and get approved for exemption, even if less than 50 people work for them. Some employers will try to coerce you out of these rights just to avoid the logistics and expense of setting this up. Several legal cases have been won when parents have been fired because an employer wanted to avoid providing these legal rights. If you are put in that position, there are organizations and lawyers that will take your case pro-bono or take their payment from winnings. Make sure you communicate everything in writing so that discrimination or unlawful firing can be proven, if needed, in court. That is why I suggest you approach this before maternity leave, as you do not want to have to go into this fight when you are postpartum and more vulnerable. If you foresee that it is going to be an issue you will have months to prepare, rather than being forced into difficult scenarios when you are more emotionally and physically vulnerable, and financially dependent on maintaining the employment.

Much of the same can be said of returning to school. You can consider trying to finish as much of your education on-line as possible to avoid some of these challenges. You might also be given access to the pump room that the school is already required to provide to its employees. Title IX also provides lactating and pregnant university students protection and ensures accommodation. Under resources there is a link to a helpful legal website with a "Breastfeeding Students" FAQs sheet for more details.

This also brings up an important aspect of pumping at work or school, and the baby needing to get bottles while you are gone. You must ensure the baby will take the bottle and that the caretaker does not overfeed the baby. It can be hard to keep up with pumping at work if your nanny keeps giving the baby 20 ounces while you are at work, but you only pump 10. It can be helpful to know what the normal intake is for your baby but does not entirely take away the risk of your baby's caretaker still overfeeding or ignoring paced-feeding advice.

Babies need about 1-1.5 ounces per hour of separation, in 3 to 5 ounce bottles every 2-3 hours. Of course, there is always variation outside of averages. I humbly suggest you meet with a lactation consultant a few weeks before going back to work to help create a plan that works for everyone. You can weigh the baby before and after feeding to see what size feed they like and avoid some of the guesswork. This kind of appointment can be extremely helpful for those who are uncomfortable giving stern and clear directions. You can then say, "the lactation consultant said only give 3 ounces, because that is what she takes from my breast," and avoid any argument based on the caretaker's expectations. You can also bring them to an appointment to have a professional explain the importance. Hopefully, they will listen. Asking your child's caretaker to help protect and preserve your breastfeeding relationship can be hard to do, especially if they do not support it or find it as important as you do. We should all be able to choose people that support us to help care for our babies, but this is sadly not the reality for many parents.

If you are having a hard time keeping up with pumping while at work, you can add pump sessions into your day elsewhere. Many parents pump after their morning nursing session, on their commute to work, on their commute home, and an extra time before bed. Fitting in extra pump sessions can be tricky and require some creativity. It is also okay to supplement if you cannot make these things work, but if you go all day most days of the week without pumping you will start to dry up. In general, you do not want to routinely go more than 3 hours between pump sessions, but the time frame that is safe can vary for each person depending on their capacity. Rather than watching the clock, feel your mammae. The more often they feel full, the more your body is getting the signal that you do not want that milk. Try to pump often enough to avoid feeling very full multiple times per day.

Benefits of breastfeeding

I will just go over briefly some of the benefits of breast-feeding that research has found, and then go into all the logistical benefits that I see outside of that. There are many great sources freely available if you wish to review all of the health benefits in detail.

For babies, the benefits include reduced risks of sudden infant death syndrome (SIDS), optimal oral palate and facial bone formation, reduced risk of childhood cancers, and an increase of antibodies that leads to reduced illness and time frame of illness. The cost of medical care for breastfed babies overall tends to be less as they get better quickly, and have less illnesses in general. For example, they tend to get less ear infections, have less diarrhea, have more regular bowel movements, have less skin issues like eczema, and the list goes on. Breastfed babies may have less instances of allergies and asthma. Having breastmilk be part of the diet helps beneficial gut bacteria to flourish, which research suggests is helpful in prevention of many chronic illnesses. Breastmilk is also less likely to be contaminated than formula. Babies who get breastmilk and formula are not really studied, but an educated guess would have me believing that all the benefits of the breastmilk are there, even if you are doing a combination of the two. These benefits are not all guaranteed, just statistically more likely, as we also have to factor in genetics, lifestyle, exposure to toxins and illnesses, and all nutritional intake.

It is beneficial that human milk is a living and changing substance. It changes to meet baby's health, nutritional, and hydration needs. It contains antibodies that fight against disease and infection. There are sugars that feed the healthy bacteria in the gut. Breast milk contains stem cells that go on to become part of the baby's body. Breast milk contains cannabinoids that encourage the baby to eat and promote neuronal development. Breast milk contains special fats that are species specific and help with brain and neurodevelopment. There are many things in breastmilk that are not in formula, and we discover more as we continue to investigate it.

For females some of the benefits are reduction of risk of several cancers like breast and ovarian, boosts of oxytocin that help regulate mood, decreased risk of osteoporosis, decreased risk of heart disease, reduced risk of stroke, diminished risk of type-2 diabetes, and many other health benefits. Many females report mental and emotional health benefits of nursing, as well. Parents also have a large financial incentive to provide breast milk over formula, as the lactating parent is often willing to provide the free labor of nursing the baby or extracting the milk. Though, a more complicated nursing relationship that needs more support than usual may end up being just as expensive or more expensive than formula feeding. Expenses can add up quickly with consults, herbs, and paraphernalia.

Society benefits at large when babies are breastfed. Breast-feeding produces less pollution and has less ecological and economic impact than formula. Overall, the healthcare system has lower costs associated with long term care of breastfed infants, and of females who have breastfed.

Psychological and mental health benefits to breastfeeding come partly from the physical boost of oxytocin but also from the feelings associated with choosing to nurse and being able to meet our baby's basic needs. Pride in yourself for your choices and for powering through the challenges, is an example. Solidarity and community with other nursing parents, are others. Social benefits extend beyond community and sometimes have unexpected perks, such as being able to leave a crowded room to nurse and thus get a break at an overstimulating social gathering.

Parenting benefits of nursing can go on for years. When

your child is facing something upsetting or is having a hard time it can be a great parenting tool to have your mammae to offer for comfort or distraction. The longer you nurse, the longer this tool is available. Additionally, with toddlers there is less worry around their solid intake. While toddler appetite waxes and wanes when it comes to solid intake you will be sure they get well balanced nutrition from their several nursing sessions throughout the day and night. Most toddlers will at least nurse twice a day, but 3 to 5 sessions may be more typical. Some still want to nurse more often than that, especially when co-sleeping with their parents throughout the night.

When you choose to exclusively breastfeed, or are able, this means less equipment to clean, use, and carry around. You will not need to lug around a pump, bottles, or formula. This is extremely helpful when you realize that you already need a lot of extra stuff to run around with a baby in tow.

Another benefit of the breast over formula is that breast milk changes as baby ages and does not continue to go up in volume throughout the year, where formula requires more and more volume to satisfy baby's needs. Breastmilk adjusts in nutritional content to satisfy baby, and changes with their gut development. Formula is not a living product like breastmilk, so it is unable to be tailored in this way to your baby. A breastfed baby might take 3 to 5 ounces or so per feeding for the entire year, where a formula fed baby needs upwards of 8 ounces per session by 6-9 months. There are some theories that this stretching of the tummy and loss of an appetite and satiety self-regulation is partially why formula fed babies might be more prone to obesity.

Another couple of periphery benefits are due to having medicine and food in your mammae, on demand. The breastmilk is readily available and easily accessible. Breast milk has stem cells and antibodies that make it ideal for helping heal minor injuries, infections, or irritations. It can help clear baby acne, help heal cracked nipples, minor rashes or infections that are not fungal, and many more practical uses. Some females use their milk in their drinks and food, for any recipes that call for milk as an ingredient. This not only would provide health benefits to those ingesting it but might also save money on buying milk at the store.

milk as an ingredient. This not only would provide health benefits to those ingesting it but might also save money on buying milk at the store.

Other People and Your Breastfeeding Relationship

Sadly, lactation is an afterthought for most healthcare providers. Most of us only get 1 to 3 hours of lactation education during school, and then never take continuing education related to lactation again. The minimum for IBCLCs to become certified is taking college level biology, anatomy, physiology, infant and child growth and development, nutrition, psychology, research, sociology, as well as 90 hours of lactation specific education, then 1000 hours of mentoring. To maintain an IBCLC there is required continuing education focused on lactation related topics and life support, documentation, terminology, occupational safety, ethics, and universal safety precautions. So, regrettably, many professionals will give you bad or outdated advice due to this huge difference in what is the necessary starting education standpoint for giving professional lactation advice. Do not assume a provider who is not also an IBCLC is up to date and wise to all current breastfeeding related guidelines, nor that they have an adequate education specific to lactation or nutrition.

Additionally, a wise provider does not ignore traditional Western Medicine and lifestyle practices due to lack of research evidence. It dishonors many cultures and Western Medicine when we discount the experience of billions of people over thousands of years. The ideal is bringing gifts from the East and West together and promoting things that are important to the family and culture, as long as they are not harmful. For example, I might not have evidence that malunggay ingestion helps boost supply, but many Asian females have had success using this galactagogue for thousands of years and there is no evidence that it is harmful. Therefore, I would find it acceptable to try if my patient so desired and would not discourage her from doing so.

Part of my job is to help keep you safe, and giving my best educated guess is required in many cases. Breastfeeding supportive professionals, in my mind, should support you and your family, because breastfeeding is a family event. Part of that is supporting and respecting social and cultural norms within your family.

Professionals are often breastfeeding tolerant but not truly breastfeeding supportive. They support it, until there is a problem. If they are truly breastfeeding supportive, they will help lead you to other professionals that can help you properly troubleshoot whatever issues are arising. Professionals are often compulsive in their needs to offer a solution when you present with a problem, and with breastfeeding that advice might be unintentionally sabotaging. It is not common for professionals to be in the habit of referring out as often as they should be. I hope to see more normalization of humility in the medical profession in the years to come. This can only serve our patients better when we defer to those with more specialty knowledge than us. Until then, as a parent you will have to be sure to seek specialty advice from those who specialize in the area you need help in. You may need to advocate for referrals or seek your own specialists.

Providers are usually guilty of suggesting you "top off" the baby with a bit of supplement without proper follow up with a lactation consultant, but many parents make this mistake on their own, too. Sometimes this is suggested because there is poor weight gain, but sometimes it is because they are dismissing true medical issues and ignoring the need for a specialty assessment or attributing normal newborn behaviors to a problem. When we top off the baby without working on protecting the supply or troubleshooting why the baby is not gaining well, then we sabotage the breastfeeding relationship by reducing the supply even further. The cycle of topping up keeps snowballing until the supply disappears. Many females get into this trap and wonder why they mysteriously dried up.

Frustration also often arises with professionals seeming to keep you on a "need to know" basis, where they decide what you need to know. Medicine in general is moving towards a more collaborative and shared-decision making model where the provider educates the patient and lets them make decisions from an informed place. I am glad to see this change, as ultimately, I believe all decisional power should be with the patient and their family. Until this cultural shift has more fully been adopted, you will inevitably face many professionals who still patronize their patients by withholding information and trying to make decisions for you.

Differences are also often perceived from one lactation consultant to the other. This is because they each have a different knowledge base, skill set, personal bias, and experience level. Not all lactation consultants are IBCLCs, and not all IBCLCs have further medical training like RNs, NPs, and MDs who serve dual roles. Often even well trained and well-meaning consultants give bad advice. Savvy IBCLCs pick up on important subtleties, regardless of education level. If you find you are not getting the support you need or you are not making progress in your care plan, it might be time to seek someone who has more experience, has more education, or is in a different specialty.

Realistically, the plan may need to change from day to day and each consultant will have the most current assessment of your breastfeeding relationship and its needs. This will feel conflicting and confusing because a new assessment and a new consultant might bring new or conflicting suggestions. Often when they suggest something different it is because the current plan is ready to progress, or it is not working well. It is okay to ask why their plan differs from the last consultant's if you are seeing more than one.

Additionally, many lactation consultants come from a place of privilege and have narrow minded ideas and limited suggestions due to their ease with their own breastfeeding experiences, including the level of support they received. Typically, a lactation consultant goes into the profession because they enjoyed breastfeeding, it went relatively well, and they had the social and economic support to make it work. They also had the support needed to obtain their education.

Another glaring issue with professionals, especially in maternal health, is that it is not completely normalized to seek consent to touch a patient. While most of us are working on developing a habit of seeking consent you will probably, more often than not, be touched without being asked. This is especially troublesome when it involves breastfeeding. It can feel very invasive and abrupt to have a stranger touch your breasts unexpectedly, and touch your infant unexpectedly. In the mind of the professional it is expected; the surprise is usually experienced by the parent. Unfortunately, in the current climate I would caution you to expect lack of asking for consent from most of your labor and delivery and postpartum team. Even though I myself am aware of the importance and need to seek consent, I sometimes forget or assume consent. If you foresee that this might be a triggering or upsetting experience, it will unfortunately require you to advocate for yourself. I do hope to see, and have started to see, a change in this behavior in the parent-infant healthcare teams and a change in the maternal health culture to remind each other to seek consent before touching another person.

Different professionals also have different personal levels of zeal for breastmilk and varied feelings about formula. Some consultants or peers who feel very strongly about breast milk only and avoiding formula at all costs put babies lives and parent's mental health in danger. If the plan the lactation consultant presents threatens either, find a new one. With all professionals it is appropriate to seek second or third opinions until the plan presented sits well with you, or even ask the professional to present alternative options. I believe a good consultant takes your goals into account and helps devise a reasonable and logical plan that will not threaten your mental health. They should also be educating you and engaging in shared decision making. Alas, we are not all created equal, nor do we have the same priorities—but there are great consultants out there who do consider you as more than just a milk machine.

Another common place that professionals will confuse you or let you down are in their assessments of your breast tissue. Many maternal health providers do not even assess your glandular tissue or discuss your breast development outside of asking if you have seen any changes during pregnancy. If you say no, they brush it off anyway. Insufficient glandular tissue (IGT) signs are often not assessed for properly or are over-looked. This leaves many parents frustrated when they are several weeks (or months) postpartum and the concept of IGT is first brought to their attention. Many professionals are advocating for this to be assessed for and brought up in prenatal or pre-conception assessments. Every pregnant person would benefit from a prenatal consult with an IBCLC, and your risks of low supply should be being discussed.

It is also no secret that there is a huge problem with racism and bias in care causing gaps in treatment in the healthcare community, especially in infant and maternal health. The statistics showing lower breastfeeding rates of black and brown babies, as well as the outpouring of women's voices calling attention to this lived experience are proof that this is a problem and change needs to happen. It is important to know that you are not being dismissed or discouraged because of your race or ethnicity when a provider has bias based on that. Many people feel most comfortable seeking IBCLCs that are the same race and ethnicity as them, but there is inequality in the ability to obtain certification, so it is not always possible. Lack of diversity in the IBCLC profession makes it a challenge for many people to find culturally or ethnically similar professionals to work with. Luckily, telehealth is more prevalent than ever, and this can open up a lot of options for people that are concerned that this might play a role in their care.

Additionally, the healthcare profession as a whole is working to train everyone to be more culturally and racially sensitive, and to root out any bias in their practice. It is also fair when you are meeting your consultants and healthcare professionals to scrutinize their approach and challenge where you suspect bias. This might present as being offered formula under the assumption you will not breastfeed or being outright discouraged from breastfeeding. A compassionate and educated provider should meet you with empathy when you challenge them, and ideally be self-aware and sensitive. If not, you can fire them and request a different caregiver. The sacred breastfeeding relationship deserves protection, especially in the black and brown communities where breastfeeding rates are lower, and infant and maternal mortality and morbidity rates are higher. You might be harder pressed to find anti-racist breastfeeding help and need to seek multiple opinions or providers. I wish it were not the reality. I am hopeful of the shift taking place in maternal-infant health that supports exposing these biases and supports bringing more black and brown providers into the maternal-infant healthcare team. I believe it is part of my duty as a healthcare provider and decent human being to call out racism, and it starts with working on myself and checking my own biases, much of which I have done over my career and will continue to do. I will also continue to encourage my peers to do the same.

Many professionals also work from a bias of what is most important to them. Often, they will not admit what is outside of their scope because they are accustomed to having all the answers. For example, Pediatricians tend to put your baby first and may be less concerned with your experience of breastfeeding, as long as your baby is gaining weight. They will be quick to blame you or your milk for a weight gain issue. An obstetrician might just encourage breastfeeding for the health benefits, while ignoring that baby is not thriving. A pediatric dentist who releases oral tethers might be more likely to release lip ties as they effect dentition and orthodontics, while an Ear Nose and Throat specialist might only revise a lip tie that is affecting breathing or nasal clearance. Then there are even fewer who will release the tie because they know it is affecting breastfeeding. The examples of these shortcomings in infant and maternal health practices are endless. Few providers look at the lactating parent and the infant as a unit, and practice holistically.

You will need to be an advocate for your child and likely step outside your comfort zone in order to find out what is best for them. You might have push-back from your pediatrician who will likely be your baby's "gate-keeper" for official referrals through insurance. This might be a good topic to ask your pediatrician about before you choose them to care for your baby. Pediatricians will often have someone they prefer you to see for specialty concerns, and that might not be the best person in town to see, but it is ultimately up to you who you take your baby to see. Go into the process as informed as possible.

All things considered, with professionals and your breastfeeding relationship, this will likely be when you learn to tap into your protective instincts and your gut instincts. An uncomfortable but necessary shift from being someone's child to then being someone's parent requires that you learn to advocate for yourself, for your child, and for your breastfeeding relationship. Many people do not realize that being a self-advocate or child-advocate in medical care is needed until it is too late. While it is good to defer to professional expertise it is also good to ask questions and challenge things that do not seem right. The best medical professionals will appreciate that you keep them on their toes.

Another issue with professionals, is that they are not always available to everyone. Lack of access to care can be a problem if you have no insurance or you are not physically near enough to a provider to make it reasonable or feasible for you to get to them, or vice versa. The "Resources" section near the end of the book has some websites that have good information such as home remedies for common issues, and links to information about legal rights for pregnant and lactating females under current healthcare laws in the USA. You might also be able to book with someone online, or search online for local help that is at no cost.

Breastfeeding and your partner

In a perfect world you will have a supportive and compassionate partner that fully joins this wild ride with you and takes everything in stride. In the intimacy of partnered heterosexual relationships, it is important to note a disturbingly common issue: a male partner might not support breastfeeding, might find it disgusting, or might also sexualize the experience. Many cultures hyper-sexualize the breast, forgetting their true intended biological purpose. This is more an issue with your partner's cultural conditioning than it is with them as a person. No need to throw the whole partner out. This might manifest as anger in a partner who is uncomfortable expressing emotion, and the underlying emotion is likely fear.

This might take some education and finesse. Ideally, you will start talking about this before you decide to have children together or during pregnancy before the baby comes. Your partner may have different levels of comfort than you with regards to how much you cover or do not cover in public, and whom you allow to see you nursing. It might take several conversations and some education to get your partner on the same page as you. Having a supportive partner is one of the top predictors of breastfeeding success, so having a physically and emotionally supportive partner is crucial. Ideally, you should sit and discuss your expectations together before the baby comes. Ask them to do the personal work around why they are uncomfortable and explore how they can support your breastfeeding success by supporting normalizing breastfeeding.

Regardless of orientation or gender, in the sexual intimacy of your relationship, being a breastfeeding parent can change a few things. This information could almost be listed as a "cost" to breastfeeding, but truly a postpartum body will need many adjustments to sexual intimacy, even if you do not breastfeed. Leaking of milk, general overstimulation, nipple tenderness, vaginal dryness, and decreased libido can be some of the things that affect you. Most of these issues can just be talked about with your partner to trouble-shoot and work around.

Most lactating females will leak milk when they have sexual relations, as the oxytocin that boosts with pleasure also increases with nursing and milk let-down. Leaking may turn your partner off, they may be indifferent to it, or it may turn them on. It is okay to talk and explore what you both feel comfortable doing with this new change. Wearing your bra to catch the leaking may be an option, especially if you find that you prefer your mammae be touched minimally while you are lactating. Alternatively, you may enjoy for your partner to suck on your nipple. Your partner might decline or respond enthusiastically. You should both approach options with an open mind and come to mutual agreements around each other's desires, comfort, and expectations. In sensitive conversations like this you will hopefully both feel heard and respected. These are not discussions to be had in the heat of the moment, but when you can both feel safe and vulnerable with each other. You will also need to consider that you will have varying degrees of personal comfort, breast soreness, and nipple tenderness, and might just take it on a case by case basis.

Hormonal changes to the reproductive organs that we discussed previously also play a part in changes to your intimate relationship. The vaginal dryness that is caused by lack of estrogen when nursing can make for painful penetrative sex. Please, use lubrication and start slow and gently with some foreplay (even if you have not needed it before). It is best to wait until about 6 weeks after delivery to try to have sex, to minimize risk of uterine infection. Your body still recovering from delivery might make sexual acts painful, or leave you feeling self-conscious about how your body is so different. Hormonal changes may also suppress your sexual desires, as breastfeeding suppresses ovulation in most females. Discomfort during penetrative sex often goes on months beyond the 6-week clearance to try, especially if you had bad tearing, so be patient. When females do not ovulate, they usually do not have periods. Often nursing parents experience period like symptoms without bleeding. For many females, the period cycle does not return or is irregular while breastfeeding. This suppression of ovulation and thus decreased desire is nature's way of encouraging greater spacing between children to allow your body time to heal, replenish stores of nutrition, and give your nursling milk for an optimal time frame. Without ovulation you do not have the ebbs and flows of hormones that make you extra aroused around ovulation, and the generally suppressed estrogen influences your over-all desire.

Additionally, the sleep deprivation can make that extra 15 minutes to spare seem like it should only be made available to sleep through, and you would never consider spending it being sexually intimate. The sheer exhaustion and work load of parenthood can make it hard to have time to get in the mood, you might be consumed with fear of pregnancy, and you might find yourself resenting your partner rather than wanting to jump their bones. You might experience guilt around wanting to be sexually intimate less often, or your lack of libido.

Breastfeeding and general partner intimacy can be challenging because care-takers of young children often feel "touched out" and overstimulated from having another body attached to them 10 hours a day. Amplify that if you have multiple children. You will have less time and energy for your partner than usual. Not just from nursing but from how physically demanding and time-consuming caring for an infant is. This will be why it is important to have a partner who chooses to take an active parenting role, or one who can be encouraged and persuaded to do so.

Now, some people might argue that you should not have to teach or encourage your partner how to help you or how to be a parent, but this is just not reality. I wish it were true that our culture turned out partners that were equalitarian in parenting, but until that day arrives, we have to work with what we have. Many partners, regardless of gender, are not prepared for the logistical demands of parenting a newborn. Even when we know what to do, many of us have engrained cultural messages about how all of the work should fall to the female parent. Many partners also lack confidence and are afraid of messing up.

It can help strengthen your relationship to set clear expectations as to how much help you expect, and with what things. Expecting your partner to know or to read your mind will probably just leave you feeling resentful and frustrated. Your partner likely assumes you just want to handle it all yourself or is afraid of interfering or insulting you by helping. You will not know until you talk about it. You cannot assume they will help, or know how to, unless you ask. Most of our partners are not abusive jerks who wish to benefit off exploiting our efforts and are happy to help if you just tell them what you expect.

From the partner's perspective they may struggle with feeling incompetent, feeling left out, and feeling unprepared. Many partners report feeling jealousy towards the baby, who is now getting to be on your breast frequently not only getting physical affection but also your attention. They may struggle with understanding the effort you put into breastfeeding if they do not find it as important as you. Conversely, they may find breastfeeding more important than you do and put pressure on you to succeed or make decisions that are not best for your mental health. Open conversations around how you are both processing things, what you are feeling, and what you are expecting will be critical to the health of your relationship. It may be hard to not become emotional or easily upset when you are hormonal and vulnerable. This is why these conversations are better handled before the baby comes, but it is never too late to have them.

Remind each other often that this is temporary. You can find new and creative ways to be intimate and connect in the quiet moments. You can find a new strength in this role as parents, partners in a new, exciting, and important phase in your lives. You will likely need to lean on your family and friends, or get creative, in order to help you to find time to connect with each other away from the new demands and stresses of parenthood.

There will be gifts and growth in your relationship as you navigate these challenges. Many couples make the mistake of thinking this turbulence during this time means they are not meant to be together, when in fact it is a normal part of relationship growth. When we face the challenges together and learn to lean in and grow together, we come out of it stronger and more connected. It is a time where you will redefine your relationship and it invites discussions, opens old wounds, and attracts change. You may fall in love all over again as you see how much your partner loves your baby. You might find yourself triggered by some of their parenting behaviors. It will be critical through this time to communicate very openly, work together, and remind each other often that you are still a team, and that you can get through this together.

Alternatively, this may be the first time you see that your partner was not who you expected and they are not willing to step up to be that, to compromise, or to grow with you. To leave out that this phase of life can cause the dissolution of relationships would be a disservice. For all the opportunities of growth are also chances of disconnect, and not every relationship survives moving into a partnership of parenthood.

If a person is with an abusive partner, pregnancy and breastfeeding often exacerbate and escalate the abuse. People who are in an abusive relationship have to consider many concerns. If they are remaining in the relationship, they might not breastfeed if their partner is not supportive, for fear of violence or other abuse, or because their partner ridicules and harasses them about it. The period of pregnancy and lactation make the abused more vulnerable and often make abusive partners more insecure, so they lash out more. If a person decides to leave based on these changes, they still have to consider economic resources, housing, custody, social support, legal help, and navigating the logistics of the legal system. Steering through all of this on top of learning to be a parent plus trying to maintain a breastfeeding relationship can feel impossible. If you find yourself in this situation know that help is available and it is possible to leave, and to be safe. My "resources" section will have more information on where and how to obtain help.

If you start a new partnership or romance, or if you start dating then the challenges can be everything we just covered, plus navigating a new relationship. There are people who seek to date lactating or pregnant partners because it is a turn on for them, so it can be hard to distinguish if your new partner is looking to establish a relationship or is seeking temporary indulgence. Dating with children could be an entire other book, so I will just stop there.

Breastfeeding and other people you live with

If you are a person that lives with an extended or blended family, you might give more thought to your choices around breastfeeding at home than someone who lives alone or with only their partner. If you live with older children, you might also pause to reflect. Creating an open dialogue about your expectations of each other before the baby comes can be helpful in navigating this change in dynamic around the house. It might require awkward and forward conversations with stepchildren, in-laws, co-parents, grandparents, or anyone who might be impacted or have an opinion. In this context, when I say people you live with, I also mean friends and family that are around very frequently such as several times a week, or most days.

Many modern families are blends of several families and thus several cultures. The cultural expectations can be different in each family micro-culture, just as it is often different from one larger culture to another. It is not unreasonable to begin to explore your family's ideals, opinions, and expectations around breastfeeding. Hopefully, you will all be able to see eye to eye on breastfeeding plans. If not, it will be harder to navigate when you are already actively breastfeeding. Sometimes your parents or your in-laws may want you to breastfeed more than you do. In many cultures and religions, breastfeeding is expected and insisted upon. If you do not meet this expectation, they might insinuate that you are lazy or a bad parent. Sometimes they expect you to leave the room or cover your baby and breast. These are not things that you want to find out or be pressured about when you are feeling your most vulnerable in the postpartum period.

Discussions often go best when you go in with an open mind and without the intention of changing other people's minds. It can take several discussions to come to new agreements that keep breastfeeding from being a point of contention amongst family. Many parents find that after several discussions they feel it is best to just avoid the family members that cannot be flexible about breastfeeding expectations, at least until after they are done nursing. Agreements and compromises cannot always be made, especially with some things such as breastfeeding. People tend to have strong opinions about it.

If the family you live with hyper-sexualizes breasts, they might be highly offended at the idea of you nursing around the house and expect you to hide in your room or wean prematurely. You may have stepparents or co-parents of the children you live with that would like you to avoid nursing around their children. The earlier in pregnancy that you approach the subject and try to normalize the expectation that you will be nursing, the easier the change will be. Be prepared that you may not come up with a solution that makes everyone happy, and you might have to just make decisions that work for you and your baby. Ultimately, it is not up to the others what you do with your own body.

Sometimes the people who are close to you know nothing about breastfeeding, and their assumptions and comments can be frustrating or hurtful. Family members who formula fed may question how you know your baby is getting enough, or still believe that formula is superior to breastmilk because that is what they were told when they were having babies. They might suggest you are selfish for breastfeeding, or say you are a bad parent for not giving formula. Sometimes parents and grandparents can take your decision to breastfeed, when they formula fed, as a personal insult. When we make different parenting decisions than them, they might perceive this to mean that our judgement of them is that they made the wrong choice when they chose something else. When these insecurities or negative assumptions go unaddressed, they might show up in other ways, such as negative commentary about breastfeeding. If you suspect or know that this is creating tension within your tribe, it is best to address it head on. Simply explaining that you are doing what you think is best for your child, just like they did, might put it in a new perspective for them. You might need to set boundaries with these people if a frank discussion does not dissuade them from making rude comments and say that this topic is no longer up for discussion any time they bring it up. For some parents this has made a temporary break from certain family members necessary.

If you have an older child, especially a toddler, expect some questions. Your toddler might try to nurse even if they weaned or never nursed because they have a biological instinct to do so. You might find they are more interested in your mammae, even in pregnancy. They sense and smell the milk. If you let them attempt to latch, they will likely not know how to draw out milk and not ask to try again. Their curiosity and desire to nurse also stems from wanting to know that you would be willing to nurture them in the same way you do their sibling. Some toddlers do resume nursing in tandem with their new sibling, and a parent might nurse them both for a while.

Older children tend to just accept the new normal with a simple explanation. It can be as easy as explaining that baby humans drink from female human's mammae, just like puppies drink from the female dam dog's teats. You might decide you feel more comfortable covering your breasts when they are present, but know that not doing so just helps normalize the breast as a non-sexual body part and normalizes the act of feeding the child from the breast. Children, even older ones, will often just follow your lead. If you make the breast to be a sexual and hidden part of the body, then that is what they will reconcile it as in their mind. If you promote it as just a normal part of the cycle of life and teach them to expect to see mammae in a non-sexual way, then they will quickly adjust.

Breastfeeding and your relationship with yourself

In many ways the journey into parenthood is an identity crisis. Your brain is changing and molding. Your body is changing. The physical space you share with your child and being touched physically increases exponentially. You are learning on the job how to act and react in an infinite number of new ways in your new role as a parent. You are re-born, in a way. In many ways this is empowering and joyous, but any period of transition comes with some turbulence.

Breaks will be few and far between. Building a village and asking for help will be critical to your mental health. This might come in the form of social programs, charities, church connections, peer groups, friends, and family. If you are going through this journey as a single parent, this can feel daunting. Even partnered parents struggle with this, as most of the parenting load usually falls to the parent that carried and feeds the child.

It is also a struggle to navigate this time if you have lost your mother or choose not to have contact with her. This is true with the absence of a father, as well. However, it tends to be a deeper primal wound for mothers who are learning to mother without their own mother present. It can be tempting in your vulnerability to reach out to toxic parents that are still alive, and ask them for help or guidance. It is common to have feelings of anger and resentment for a mother that has died, because you wanted her here for these moments, especially to offer her guidance. The absence of a parent or parents when you are transitioning to a parental role can be very upsetting and influence your self-esteem around succeeding in your goals. The physical presence of our parents as a comfort is an engrained biological response, so their absence might leave you longing for them. The grief around these circumstances usually surfaces when we are freshly postpartum and most vulnerable, but might show up again and again as we wish we could talk and connect to share the experience and swap stories. Because child-rearing is so emotional and so hard, it is only natural to want to connect with a parent and let them be involved in the process. You may want to seek a mothering or nurturing relationship with an elder who has breastfed before in order to fulfil that role for you, because it can be very helpful to the emotional burdens of breastfeeding.

Many parents feel the strain of wanting to do it all, but not being physically able. The invisible load of parenthood asks us to handle too many things simultaneously than is good for our mental health. Learning to quiet the lies that "you are screwing up," "you aren't trying hard enough," "you are going insane," "you are inadequate," "others are succeeding more easily," will be part of some of the challenges you face. You will tackle conflicting advice, have conflicting emotions, have a hard time asking for help, and sometimes feel like you are failing. For some of us, the challenge with asking for help is a trauma response. You might struggle with feeling like you go days without getting anything done because you are consumed with exhaustion and busy with care-taking. The secret is, parenting is getting something done. This is a hard shift for people who are task oriented and accustomed to having a clean house. The same 5 tasks repeated 20 times per day can make you feel stuck or less productive. It can help to focus your thoughts on the fact that those repeated tasks add up to an exponential sum; the task of raising and loving a whole human being. There are not more important tasks. That is the most important work. It is okay to have a messy house for a while, and to let other people help you. Do not try to do it all, especially not alone. Growth and learning in this phase looks very messy, figuratively and literally. It will be ok to not feel ok, and to experience some growing pains.

You might find yourself sabotaging the help that is offered. Insisting your way is the only way. Interrupting your rest to make sure things are being done to your standards. Avoiding asking for help because explaining how to do it "right" is exhausting. You might find yourself not trusting other caregivers. These are normal responses when you are tapping into your protective role of a parent, and you will have to actively push this aside so you can get the rest you need and deserve. This is just one way where you can take the opportunity to grow and learn to trust that the people who are offering to help might do it differently, but the end result will be similar or the same. If you trust that your helper will keep your baby safe, go rest. Do not fret over details. Rested parents who have a sense of balance in their life often have more success with supply, and with continuation of breastfeeding.

You might find yourself needing to reach out for mental health help when you have never had to before. You might struggle with things you never imagined you would struggle with. This is nothing to be ashamed of or hide, and there will be resources available when you are ready. The challenge of self-regulating your reactions can be extremely hard, especially when parenting triggers trauma from your childhood. You will be called to create your new identity as a parent, and many people want to incorporate some of their own parents' habits, while leaving behind what they felt was damaging to them. This is a tall order when you are under the physical demands of parenting an infant and toddler.

You will establish a new facet of your identity, to add to your many others. You will learn to connect with and know who you are as a parent, and what that means to you. It often influences and changes the other parts of you, because… how could it not? You will likely get in touch with your inner warrior, as you learn to protect and advocate for your baby, or yourself. Being pushed to new limits can help you learn to establish boundaries more firmly. You may connect differently to your inner lover, as you now more deeply relate to the female power to bring forth life. You will likely develop an amazement and appreciation for all that your body can do. Many facets of your personality are likely to change and adapt. You will lose your old self and find your new self. Growing into this role can feel empowering and beautiful, and still be messy and scary.

Breastfeeding and your friendships.

Great friends generally support each other in their choices. However, just like your partner can be socially conditioned to find breastfeeding to be gross or sexual, so can your friends! Some of your friends may have deep trauma about breastfeeding not working out for them and they might project that pain onto you and your breastfeeding choices. They may choose to avoid you to avoid being confronted with their feelings. Friends who have never had children may also avoid you for a multitude of personal reasons. They may be sad they do not have a baby yet, they may be happy for you but do not care to be around babies, or they might feel awkward about any chance of seeing your mammae. This may come across as negative and as judgement for your choices; you may even perceive it as rejection. Remember, these are their own issues and often not a reflection of their affection for you. You may need to make more effort than you are accustomed to in order to maintain friendships, allow those friends more space and compassion, or choose to let the friendship go. Some of your friends will be your biggest supporters, and start coming around more often. Breastfeeding and your new social circles might lead you to developing new and different friendships. You will likely find you want to only make space for deep and meaningful friendships once you are a parent, and some of your friendships will fizzle out. It is not uncommon for your circle of friends to evolve or change after becoming a parent.

Breastfeeding and all the other people in the world

One of the most prevalent issues for the modern parent is the thief of joy that is social media. We spend far too much time comparing ourselves to celebrities, influencers, friends, and acquaintances. They do not share their struggles publicly, so we assume they are doing well or doing better than us. This is especially an issue in breastfeeding culture. Often a parent will want to make a social media post when breastfeeding is going well and looks easy and beautiful, or they will want to brag about their extra milk supply. They share this because they are proud, but often leave out the struggle it took to achieve it. This is not so much a character flaw as it is just human nature to want to focus on the positive outcomes and milestones. The issue is that it normalizes the idea that breastfeeding should be more peaceful, intuitive, and not much of a struggle. Do yourself a favor and avoid accounts that make you feel "less than." It can help if you try to find uplifting accounts, especially of those who will share the raw truth and the struggle, so that you feel less alone and isolated. If you need to protect yourself from social media, do it. Get totally off of it and go read a book or watch a show.

The other glaring issue with social media is the ease of peer to peer advice. While having peer to peer advice can be invaluable, it has also caused delays in seeking professional help when it was really needed. The advice offered from a professional versus a peer will include knowing your medical history and details important to treatment suggestions, and you deserve personalized and thorough care. It is too easy for people online to pretend to have credentials that they do not. Someone who is gifted with words and writing can be convincing, but that does not mean they are right. What worked for one dyad might be disastrous for another. Following the global pandemic of 2020, most professionals are available at least part time in an online platform. In the USA we are also entitled to lactation benefits through insurance. This, I think, will make care more accessible and allow parents to seek professional help when needed. If you are ever in doubt or need guidance, I would suggest using peer to peer suggestions in conjunction with professional advice, not in place of.

On social media and out in the general public, you may face mean spirited or even well-intentioned people that will shame you for however you are feeding your child. Sometimes a well-intentioned person thinks they are informing you for the first time that "breast is best" and you must not have known, since you are bottle feeding. Parents often experience things like this, the underlying message being they should be breastfeeding and not giving the baby a bottle. They will not even bother to ask if the bottle has breastmilk or formula in it. That same parent might be shamed for breastfeeding in public the very same day. People can be alarmingly rude or aggressive, in person and on the internet. Social media comments on public posts might say conflicting things from one comment to the next. Some will praise your breastfeeding; others will tell you it is gross. Remember that those who seek to shame you or unintentionally shame you have their own issues around breastfeeding or formula feeding that they have not sorted out. Normal and healthy people do not care to bother parents feeding their young, regardless of the method. Their comments say nothing about you, but a whole lot about them. Often those who comment are perpetuating myths or partial truths, so don't take them to heart.

There are so many myths surrounding breastfeeding, even in the healthcare community. Your providers, in fact, may be victim to buying into some of the myths. Several prevalent myths are repeated to new parents by their baby's well-meaning pediatricians. A common myth is that your milk is causing basically any issue with the baby. Usually it is issues that they have no explanation for, nor have they thoroughly investigated a cause for. Often colic, the witching hour, and the period of purple crying are blamed on breastfeeding or the milk itself, when really babies can have (and do have) many periods of un-explained crying for the first few months of life. Sometimes they cry so much it makes you start to lose your grip on your sanity, but that does not mean something is wrong with your milk or with your parenting. Soothing techniques should be explored before blaming the breastmilk, and there are a lot out there. Some basic soothing techniques might be returning to skin to skin to reset, shushing, swaying, nursing, going to a dark room, taking a warm bath, going for a walk in the stroller, or taking a drive in the car seat.

That being said, if your mama intuition thinks that your baby is crying excessively or is in pain, it is okay to push for answers. If your nerves are so fried from your baby constantly crying and you are not sure if its intuition or desperation, push for answers anyway. Your baby can be tested for food intoler-ances and allergies, can be assessed for tongue ties, and evalu-ated for reflux. Do not be afraid to advocate for your baby or insist on further assessment or second opinions (or third, or fourth). If soothing is not working, if the crying is excessive, if your baby might be in pain do not just push through and suffer. There should be thorough and extensive assessment and testing and multiple specialists being consulted if your baby is crying so much that it is making you worry.

Another place to lay blame that stems from a myth may be suggesting that poor weight gain for baby is from "not enough calories or fat" in your milk. Unfortunately, we know from stud-ies in time of famine that breastmilk is always made pretty perfectly. Our biological design is to place preference on our off-spring's survival. Our milk will be made from our skin and bones before it is made poorly for baby. Breastmilk should be tested before officially being blamed, and all other causes ruled out as well.

They may also suggest gastrointestinal discomfort in baby is caused by the food you eat "contaminating" your milk. Unless a food allergy has been diagnosed, this is probably not true. You will be told to "pump and dump" for many things that you do not actually need to dump milk for. You will be told to avoid foods that you do not actually need to avoid. Someone will inevitably suggest you toughen your nipples while pregnant by roughing them up with a washcloth, or tell you to wash your nipples between feedings; neither of which is necessary nor helpful. The myths and misconceptions are boundless.

For matters of breastmilk and lactation it is best to seek an IBCLC. For the general health of a baby, the pediatrician is your go-to. For special circumstances about your baby's health, you will seek a specialist such as a gastrointestinal provider. The best approach is a team approach, with multiple providers being consulted for their expertise.

Breastfeeding medicine is a specialty and deserves to be referred to just like the gastroenterologist. We all have knowledge and gifts to share that make up a successful health-care team. I would hope you find a pediatrician that is wise to their limited knowledge and comfortable saying, "Go see lactation for that!"

Another myth many parents fall prey to is hearing that their baby will not get sick if they are breastfeeding. This often leads to very frustrated parents when their baby gets their first stomach bug, cold, or ear infection. What breastmilk actually does is provide antibodies so that illnesses will have weaker symptoms and shorter than usual duration.

Nosy Nancies are what I call people that believe they need to tell you how, what, when, where, and why about breastfeeding. This can make breastfeeding in front of others, frankly, annoying. From a stranger in public to a well-meaning mother or aunt; everyone has advice. They have advice whether or not you ask for it! They have advice about many other topics, other than feeding, too! It starts with feeding, then they get into sleeping arrangements, offering solids, using car seats, potty training, vaccinating, and the list goes on.

I find responding with gratitude and following up with confident and firm boundaries helps keep these people from repeatedly suggesting the same things over and over again. I might say something like "Thank you for sharing that, I am sure you are saying it because you care very much for me and the baby, and want what is best for us. At the same time, I have done my due diligence on finding out the most updated information on this topic, and I have consulted our healthcare providers, and what we are doing is safe and is working for us. If I change my mind or want to discuss it again, I will let you know." You can practice saying something like that, but in your own words so that it feels natural and true. If this does not work, you can switch to a more direct statement to set the boundary, such as, "This topic is not up for discussion, and I am set in my decision" and then change the subject. If they still persist, it might be time to set physical boundaries and stay away from that person for a while.

For all the ways in which you parent, you might face some social stigma or criticism on social media, just as you might in person. This is not guaranteed, as some parents never experience this, but it happens often enough, that we should not ignore it. Parents who bottle feed might be told "breast is best" by strangers, or be asked, "why are you not breastfeeding?" Conversely, breastfeeding parents might be approached and told "you should have just pumped and given a bottle," or "you are not making enough to keep him full, offer a bottle of formula." You have to grow a thick skin when you become a parent and learn to tune nosy and rude people out. These comments are usually not reserved only for feeding methods but extend to every parenting decision you can make. It can make it seem like there are double standards, no good choices, and no good answers. This is obviously not true, and unless you are making unsafe choices, they are probably not worth inviting discussion.

Part of the reason so many people have conflicting information about infant feeding is due to the fact that formula companies did a great job perpetuating myths about breastfeeding and formula. They spent decades and millions convincing many people that formula was superior to breastmilk, and that only poor people breastfed. This was a global effort and is still a strong held belief in some communities. This is why many people will suggest you just give a bottle, and not understand why you fight so hard to succeed at breastfeeding.

Many others will probably offer to give bottles or wonder why you do not give bottles. Some will want to help you and want to take turns feeding the baby, arguing they need to do so to bond with baby. There are other ways to bond like baths, cuddles, swaddles, rocking, and diaper changes. But it is also okay if your long-term plan includes a bottle or two a day, you just have to pump 1-2 times per day to cover that missed stimulation. Honestly, if you have an adequate supply, many parents have successfully given breastmilk and formula for the first year just to take the pressure off of one person being the sole nutrition provider for the infant. Whatever your plan or comfort level, work with an IBCLC to ensure you can meet your long-term goal if these changes to the biological norm are introduced.

This leads me to the myth that you should completely avoid pumping and bottles the first 6 weeks, at all costs. I believe this is a somewhat fair instruction for parents who will never be separated from their infant and do not plan to let others help or do not plan to return to work. Pumping and bottle feeding from the beginning will not ruin your breastfeeding relationship if balanced right. Furthermore, if this is what parenting choice you desire then you should be given information on how to most safely do this without sabotaging your over-all goals.

I think having this as a blanketed rule just creates room for confusion when new parents are told they need to pump within the first six weeks due to breastfeeding not going well. Having this blanket rule has caused parents to ignore the advice to start pumping when it was warranted, because this rule was drilled into their brain. You need to know that there is flexibility here, and while it is ideal to biological norms it is not going to derail your entire breastfeeding journey if you have flexibility; additionally, you may be instructed to start pumping to help get more milk to the baby if they are not feeding well, or to boost your supply.

Speaking of the "no bottles" rules, that brings to mind pacifiers. The main concerns are that there will be nipple confusion, and you will miss feeding cues. Every time a baby is suckling on a pacifier that is a missed opportunity to be at the breast building supply and connection. You should be safe if you use discretion with pacifiers. Give it after or between feeds or when you need a moment to prepare to feed, and do not ignore the need to cluster feed. Your baby has a strong desire to suckle frequently, and this works in tandem with your mammae needing to have frequent stimulation, so it is not a suitable substitute for the breast more than sparingly a few times a day for the first few weeks. Examples of appropriate times to use it briefly might be while you are driving, during medical procedures, or the lactating parent is held up momentarily in the shower or going to the restroom. Many babies do well without ever having had one, and using one is mostly just a parenting choice.

Often, I find parents and professionals want to blame the pacifier for "nipple confusion" because the baby stops latching well, and usually this is a quick and effortless way to avoid thoroughly investigating why the baby will not latch. It is usually not the pacifier's fault, and it is because the baby is unhappy at the breast due to lack of flow or lack of ability to draw out milk. If your baby is refusing your breast you need an IBCLC's help, not to avoid pacifiers. Short term judicious use might be indicated, and sometimes pacifiers are used in suck-training therapy to help babies strengthen the muscles they use to breastfeed. The most recent systematic analysis of pacifier use by the World Health Organization in 2016 found that there was not a statistically significant difference in breastfeeding success at 3 months postpartum for dyads that used pacifiers from the first few days on, versus those that did not. Studies have also shown that pacifier use reduces the risk of SIDs.

You also want to consider the pacifiers effect on oral health, dental health, and speech. When you do not wean a baby off of a pacifier by 1 year, you risk issues in these developments. Sucking on bottles and pacifiers should ideally stop around one year, so that the child can learn to use their oral muscles properly, and their palate and teeth are not molded into problematic forms. It is also more challenging to convince a toddler to give up a pacifier, than an infant. Also, keep in mind using a pacifier sets you up to have to fetch it frequently when it falls out of your baby's mouth, sometimes several times a night during sleeping times. While they can be a helpful tool, they do have their downsides. Many children never take a pacifier, though, and if you never start with one you will not have to worry about the downsides. It is not mandatory that a child use one.

Expanding further on this important topic of pacifiers, is important you are not buying into the lie that your baby will use you as a pacifier. Let me make this clear, the pacifier was invented to replace the breast, not the other way around. The pacifier interrupts the biological design, but that does not make it evil. Every time you let your baby suckle at the breast you are providing multiple benefits to both yourself and your baby. They are driven to suckle as much as possible and that is not on accident. It is part of the design of the symbiotic parent-infant relationship. It helps your baby feel connected, cared for, and trusting. It helps the baby's face and palate develop optimally. It helps the postpartum body recover and boosts emotional health. That being said, this is where your discretion and best judgement will come in. It is likely a reasonable choice and low risk option to use the pacifier sparingly when the nursing parent cannot safely offer her breast or is temporarily unavailable. Examples might be while driving in the car, or when the parent is showering.

Also, remember how I said it was normal for babies to cry a lot, wake frequently, spit up a lot, poop a lot, and have a lot of gas? Many people will want to blame your milk for these normal newborn behaviors as if they are a problem. The behaviors are not a problem, the expectation of newborn bodies to function like adult bodies is the problem! These same people will often blame your breastfeeding relationship for the reason your newborn seems to need you so frequently. They will blame the fact that you are breastfeeding on the child's frequent and cumbersome physical needs. We need to stop trying to mold babies to our (often misguided) expectations, and just respond to their needs as they present them. They are, after all, little baby animals that know nothing other than instincts and needs. We cannot go wrong following their lead. Babies are learning that they can trust you with every interaction. They are learning that you will meet their needs, physical and emotional. Responding to their demands consistently and quickly creates trust and leads to a secure, independent, and well-adjusted child.

A common concern parents have around baby noises is how much they hiccup. Much like they do in-utero, they seem to spend a lot of time hiccupping the first few weeks. There are theories around the diaphragm getting more exercise after birth, causing some spasming which leads to the hiccup noise. There are also theories around the frequent hiccups ensuring that the baby keeps breathing. Many parents wonder if it is something they are doing (such as over-feeding) causing this, or if there is something they can do to help it. A few anecdotal reports of parents say letting the baby drink soothes them, just like we might drink some water to stop them. Overall, hiccupping frequently has no real known cause or pattern, and is just another normal newborn behavior. The frequent hiccups for the first few weeks do not seem to bother them or cause them pain.

As an aside, I will mention another common newborn noise that worries most parents and that is a whistle in the nose. It can sometimes sound like babies are stuffed up, but really it is just their body getting used to air and dust particles. The first few weeks they make little stuffy whistles through their nose, and its especially worse if you have a winter baby due to the heaters drying them out. This topic is kind of breastfeeding adjacent because a common cure is dripping a few drops of breastmilk into the nares. Saline sprays and drops are also sold commercially for the same purpose.

Another common myth is also that larger babies need more milk than a parent can provide, and formula will be an absolute must. In reality, newborns are needy little creatures, no matter what size they are or how you feed them. Very large babies are usually so large and thriving due to what their parent's body provides for them, so interrupting that can sabotage what good thing they have going on.

As a breastfeeding parent, others might blame your baby's frequent need to connect with you on the breastfeeding bond. Truthfully, babies should be very bonded and connected with their main caretaker and having frequent needs goes on through toddlerhood, so it is misguided that some people are bothered by it. It is a survival instinct and critical to human development that infants be near a responsive caregiver most of the time. Often babies want to be held near constantly, for much of the first 2 years of their life. High needs babies might never want to be away from an adult's touch or interaction. They are not manipulating you, and you are not spoiling them. You are both following biological norms and instincts that benefit both of you in many ways, such as psychological and physical. Baby wearing can be extremely helpful when you are having a hard time with balancing baby holding with getting tasks done. After learning about comfortable baby-wearing and doing so safely, you can then learn to nurse while baby wearing and achieve next-level parenting! Baby carriers enable many parents to get more chores done and run errands with less stress.

When babies go through the normal developmental change known as separation anxiety around 9 to 12 months of age many people like to blame a breastfeeding relationship for it. During separation anxiety the baby has a heightened sense of fear of anyone other than their main 1-2 caregivers, and they want to be held more than usual. When infants start to struggle with being separated from their main caregivers around this stage, they can use their voice and body language to protest a separation. Babies who are not breastfed go through the same phase.

Many ill-informed but well-intentioned people will also often perpetuate a myth that it is bad to let your baby nurse to sleep. This is biologically normal and how they are designed to be comforted into sleeping. The slowing of the milk flow as the breast drains and the surge of feel-good hormones during nursing helps them to relax and lull into a sleeping state. They all eventually fall asleep without the breast, so there is no need to rush stopping this practice; it is not a bad habit. Forcing or pushing babies out of this instinct results in tears on both sides. As your baby gets older, they will start napping without nursing to sleep first, and eventually go to bed without nursing to sleep.

Random people will also believe they have the cure to boost your supply, especially people that sell lactation cookies. It is important that you work with someone who knows your medical history, because supply boosting techniques are not "one size fits all." This is especially true with herbal remedies, as they work to influence hormones. Even lactation consultants are guilty of working outside their scope with herbs. Ideally, a naturopath or herbalist is who should help you find a personalized and safe herbal plan. Most commercial boosting products work by increasing the water volume and do not always work to increase enough of the nutritional content. They are best saved for when you get dehydrated from an illness or need a temporary boost when your period returns.

Realistically, when people you love and trust start telling you there is a problem with your milk or a problem with breastfeeding, you might start to believe them. Even if it does not cause you to doubt yourself, it can be frustrating and annoying. It is easier to ignore strangers. Do not let their lack of education and inexperience with newborns deter you, even if it someone you love and trust. Do not let self-doubt creep in. If you are questioning any of these baby behaviors—call in a professional to assess what is happening! Many times, the expectation of the adults needs managed, not the baby's behaviors. As babies are little animals, they are living off of just following instincts, one after the other, and they are often not leading us the wrong direction. Adults who are misinformed or over-thinking (including ourselves) are the ones who interfere and mess with nature. We need to stop asking babies to not follow their instincts, and learn to trust our babies, trust our bodies, and trust the process.

Other myths that people might try to perpetuate involve your postpartum body. Remember we went over how breast-sagging often gets blamed on breastfeeding? Well other things that are normal in a postpartum body often get blamed on breastfeeding hormones, too. One example might be when you are 3-6 months postpartum and a lot of your hair starts falling out. This can be very scary but is totally normal. When you are pregnant you do not shed as much hair and it often feels thicker. After pregnancy you shed that extra hair, and then some. Another myth others might bring up is why you are not losing weight if you are breastfeeding. This would be a good time to remind them that your body is storing fat in case of famine, so that you can still use your superpower of making milk.

Breastfeeding can also be made challenging by the many societal expectations and norms that sabotage the breastfeeding relationship. These include things like being expected to leave your nursing infant with someone else for appointments and court proceedings, as well as returning to work when they are still nursing. Another example is the varied perceptions and responses to nursing an infant in public. Cultural sabotage comes in the form of lack of legal support and protection of the preservation of the nursing relationship. These examples extend from judges giving a nursing infant custody to a non-nursing parent, up to lack of maternity leave legislation. This of course varies based on which country you live in.

People will always create judgements in their mind around your choices or needs, and some even share them out loud. Do not let that get to you. Most people mind their own business.

Not Lactating, or Not Exclusively Giving Your Own Milk

Redefining breastfeeding success

I mentioned before that breastfeeding is not an "all or nothing" game. If you face challenges, your breastfeeding goals do not have to be thrown out—just redefined. Rather than focusing on a full supply, you might need to focus on how many months (or years) you would like to breastfeed. Rather than focusing on breastfeeding, you might need to make pumping goals. Do not worry if you need gadgets to help you, or you do not make enough; that is not failure. Failure comes from my end. If I do not provide you with all the information, if I do not support your goals; I am failing you. The healthcare system often fails parents by not making an IBCLC part of all prenatal and postpartum healthcare teams, and by not making being evaluated by one a part of your routine of care. So, the responsibility may be on you to seek one out.

Benefits and challenges of formula and donor milk feeding

I would bet money you did not expect me to mention benefits of formula in a breastfeeding book! Formula is not the enemy and will not ruin your baby, your breastfeeding relationship, or their gut, or their immune system. Formula saves lives and many parents are happy to use formula and breastfeed in tandem. The same leading health authorities that promote breastfeeding also suggest using formula any time there is a medical indication. The order of preference of milk to feed infants is the biological parent's own milk from direct nursing, the parent's own milk from pumping, another person's breastmilk, and then formula. Formula would likely not exist had reasons for us to need it not existed, as necessity is the mother of invention.

In the early and fragile days while waiting for milk to come in it can keep a baby stable, especially when donor or pumped milk is not available. It can prevent babies from losing too much weight, developing brain damage from high bilirubin levels, prevent them from becoming dehydrated, stabilize blood sugar, and prevent babies from being too weak to breastfeed. It can take some of the stress off parent to be the baby's sole nutritional source. Sometimes the medical indication for formula introduction is parent's mental health. I believe this is just as important as baby's physical needs.

Having some formula in the picture also means you will not likely need to supplement with Vitamin D or iron for your baby, as it is added into formulas. Exclusively breastfed babies are at higher risk for Vitamin D and iron deficiency, and in fact Vitamin D deficiency is prevalent amongst most people. Infants, children, and adults all need extra Vitamin D, and this is a world-wide consensus. More information can be obtained from the WHO statement on Vitamin D and iron supplementation. Iron being decreased reduces baby's risk for sepsis, so it is likely low in breastmilk by biological design, but it is important for brain development. It is likely a left-over evolutionary advantageous adaptation that developed when babies used to be at higher risk for infections the first year of life. Most infants are no longer threatened with infection at the rate they were 10,000 years ago, so having enough iron for optimal brain development takes priority over keeping iron low to avoid sepsis.

You do always have the option to draw Vitamin D and iron serum levels before deciding to supplement. Many infants maintain a good iron store until they start solids at 6 months, so you could have it checked around 6 months when iron stores would start to drop. The iron in breastmilk is more bio-available for absorption than dietary iron, so its low quantity in the milk may not matter in relation to how much serum iron the baby actually has. The lower quantity in milk and the store depletion around 6 months is why you are told it is important to ensure iron rich foods are a part of the diet. Many lactating parents opt to increase their own Vitamin D supplement to get more to the baby through the milk, but this is not standard practice. This is not possible with iron supplementation, as it is not put into the breastmilk though the same process as vitamins.

Formula, pumping, and bottles have given us many gifts in our modern life but relative to the history of humans it is only very recently that we have introduced these methods of infant feeding. In many ways we are fighting thousands of years of what was normal, to try to create a new normal. Historically, females used to always be surrounded by many other lactating females. Females had many babies over their entire life, from puberty to menopause, so most of them were lactating for decades. People in general also lived in closer quarters. Villages were made of many tiny homes very close together, where we had much greater labor sharing of daily tasks. Having your friend or relative nurse your baby until your milk came in or so you could get a break was the norm. Having one person wet nurse several children so that others could focus on other jobs was the norm. Using milk from the goat or cow out back when you had low supply or had to be separated from the baby was also the norm. The human species is so flexible and resilient, and always has been!

Today, since we have pumping, bottles, and formula this gives us more options. We know that breastmilk from human parents is best for human babies; it is optimal. Yet many odds are stacked against the modern breastfeeding dyad. We live in houses, separated from our neighbors, with our small family units. You do still have the option of using a wet nurse, but it is harder to accommodate that plan in our modern lifestyles and living arrangements, unless you live in a house with multiple lactating women. If you want or need to use formula in your feeding routine, you can work with an IBCLC to maximize your supply so that you can still meet your breastfeeding goals in terms of length of time spent nursing. Many parents hybrid feed or combo feed and are able to make their long-term breastfeeding goals.

While historically understood "wet-nursing" is harder to work out logistically for most families, it is possible to do a modified version. This practice has not disappeared, it is just less common. One way it has increased in modern society is through informal peer to peer milk-sharing. Parents who pump excess milk or surrogates who do not have a baby to feed are offering their milk online and in local peer groups. Some sell it and some donate it. This practice poses risks just as formula feeding does. Making this choice, in my opinion, is like choosing which foods to feed your child. It is a parenting decision and if you choose to do so I would recommend following some safety measures.

The safest way to engage in peer to peer milk sharing would be having a donor who has been screened and verified as a safe donor. In the absence of that it is not uncommon to ask for medical records showing absence of communicable disease. Discussing intake of diet, drugs, and alcohol would be beneficial in case you have any personal objection to certain practices or need a diet specific to your child's sensitivities.

While we are discussing breastfeeding alternatives, this might be a good place to explain why most people who promote breastfeeding as optimal do not like the "fed is best" campaign. Though we can follow the logic that keeping a baby fed and thriving is better than the alternative of death, this does not negate that being fed human milk as a human child is optimal. Those who run the fed is best campaign play on emotions and semantics to promote formula feeding and bash breastfeeding. They water down or down-play the benefits of breastmilk and breastfeeding, which makes many parents believe it is not that important to try to breastfeed. Being hung up on the word "best" causes so many unnecessary arguments, when in reality most people with common sense can see that what is best is subjective. The Fed is Best campaign is accused of a desire to sabotage breastfeeding relationships and being financially backed by formula companies. Of course, there are also lactivists that swing too hard the other direction and say breast is best, full stop. I think both camps are too hung up on semantics, seeking a cute and catchy phrase for something that is more complicated and nuanced than a three-word motto can encompass.

What is really "best" is subjective to each family, and specific to their situation. I believe what is best is when a parent is informed and empowered to make decisions that work for them. I would rather see a parent who is happy and thriving choosing to formula feed, than a depressed and miserable one trying to breastfeed when they hate it.

It can also provide as an unmeasurable relief when formula is used to sustain a baby's life and help them thrive. We are clearly universally benefited by the option of formula in many ways, and it should be a part of infant feeding conversations. Many parents are empowered by formula to help their babies thrive, where they would otherwise become sickly, malnourished, or die. Most parents reading this book will have access to clean water and be able to properly sterilize their formula and bottle-feeding equipment. Some even have the luxury of choosing the best formula and bottles that money can buy.

Despite all this, it would still be unfair of me not to discuss the downsides of formula, just as I have discussed the downsides of breastfeeding. Promoting formula only or formula over breastmilk has been historically proven to cause more infant illness and death and create a greater economic burden on the healthcare system. In many countries where resources are limited, the shift to formula feeding over breastfeeding has caused many needless infant deaths. It is logistically more challenging to formula feed than breastfeed, when breastfeeding goes well. You have to stay on top of the stock of formula you have, have access to clean water, have a way to sterilize the formula, choose the best formula, find the best bottle and nipple, stay on top of cleaning bottle parts, pack more in the diaper bag, take up time to prepare a bottle, worry about constipation, and deal with negative judgements from others. You might need to trial several different formulas before you find one that your baby responds well to. While I do not believe formula is bad or evil, we cannot discuss its benefits without also considering its risks or shortcomings. It is a beautiful thing that it exists and is available, but it should not be our default. If we provide even some breast milk or do some nursing part-time, we provide all the benefits and mitigate some of the risks associated with formula feeding. Taking away even some breastmilk takes away all the benefits of the milk, the act of nursing, and lactating for both the parent and the infant. This is why truly comprehensive breastfeeding and formula education is so important. Education on one should not be without companion of education on the other.

Not Breastfeeding

Sometimes, providing breastmilk is not possible, even in small quantities or with part-time nursing. While you may be forced into not breastfeeding, some people choose not to for a myriad of personal reasons. Not breastfeeding will not affect how good of a parent you are, as you are so much more than a milk machine. Your baby gets many benefits from having a loving and connected caregiver. That, arguably, can be more important than feeding method.

Some people are faced with a cancer diagnosis while pregnant or breastfeeding. This might be breast cancer, but it may not. Chemotherapy and radiation are not compatible with breastfeeding and might necessitate you forgo breastfeeding in order to get the appropriate treatment you need. If it is breast cancer, you might have to get a mastectomy, making traditional breastfeeding an impossibility. However, after reconstruction, you might breastfeed with an SNS. If you are able to keep your breasts, it is possible to establish your milk supply and dump your milk until it is safe to start feeding baby. It is also possible to re-lactate after chemo or radiation, to bring in a supply and attempt to get baby to breast later on while in remission. It is okay if these options do not appeal to you, as it may be more appropriate to you to grieve the loss and move on, without re-visiting the option.

We touched on insufficient glandular tissue in the "low supply" section. Often this means there is no breast tissue development, and no milk ever came in beyond a few milliliters. If you experience this, you might choose not to continue nursing, or your baby may refuse the breast. If you have more children, you might choose to avoid even attempting to nurse.

We also touched on past sexual trauma influencing nursing. Sometimes the trauma is so severe that the thought of nursing is too upsetting or repulsive.

We also touched on how your body changes, and how your weight might be greater than usual. Parents with eating disorders often find this change too hard to cope with and choose not to nurse.

Illnesses or chronic diseases might cause you to need a medication that is not compatible with nursing, and you will have to choose not to in order to preserve your health, or you will decide that the risks do not outweigh the benefits. It is possible that some diseases go into remission while breastfeeding, so it is always worth investigating if yours might before making that call. Some parents in this situation will give it a 3 to 6-month trial before getting back on their medications. In that time, new medications might come out that are compatible, or you might learn that you have not tried all of the options, and that some options left are actually compatible with nursing. With the hormonal changes of pregnancy and nursing one medication that did not work for you previously might work while you are nursing.

Quitting earlier than planned for your mental health might also come up. I do not wish for you to martyr yourself to breastfeeding. Your baby needs you, the real, whole, and healthy you, more than they need breastmilk.

You do not owe anyone an explanation, no matter the reason. It is okay to choose not to breastfeed. It is okay to decide breastfeeding is not working for you. It is okay to decide the benefits are not being outweighed by the risks to your mental, physical, and emotional health. Though, some people may pry or demand explanations, you do not need anyone else in the world to understand your decision or your reasons, that is for you to know and to own.

Grieving might be a part of this process, even when you are confident in your decision. Sometimes grief comes with feeling frustrated, angry, or defeated. You will likely experience misplaced negative feelings towards people who promote breast-feeding or are proud of breastfeeding. You might find yourself perceiving some one's celebration of breastfeeding or education around breastfeeding as a slight to you, or think it is meant to be taken as a shaming statement to those who feed formula. Often, it is not the true intention of the person celebrating or educating; but grief can cloud our judgement. And when someone does intentionally shame you over it, it can wound deeply. It can take some parents years to recover from not breastfeeding, whether they felt empowered in their decision or not.

Drying up and weaning

Drying up the supply can be a challenge. This is especially taxing when you are not totally comfortable with the decision to wean. Sometimes the decision revolves around a tragedy, such as a cancer diagnosis, an infant death, or physical separation from the child. Sometimes the decision happens when a parent needs to step away from breastfeeding because they are too heartbroken over struggling with their supply, or the baby's latch. Slow and steady natural weaning elicits the same responses within us as faster and forced weaning. Weaning from pumping can trigger the same changes as weaning from feeding on the breast. Even when it is a clear and definitive choice, your hormones and biological drives will make it hard to do. Mammae want to lactate and feed all the babies and they will resist drying up.

In the early postpartum days, the milk will always come in initially for most females, and they will likely experience engorgement pain. This is also true even if a baby does not survive; it can happen after a miscarriage or infant demise. If this happens the healthcare team can discuss strategies for comfort as well as herbal and supplemental remedies to help aid the process. If the milk is persistent one can discuss medication options with their provider.

One can also schedule with a lactation consultant if they decide they would like to encourage milk production at that time, or later in the future if they decide they want to bring it back again. The more recent it has been since weaning, the easier it can be to re-lactate.

If drying up after having nursed for some time (weeks or months), one would have to stop gradually. Slowly spacing out feedings or pump sessions is best. An abrupt stop to milk removal creates a high risk for clogs and mastitis.

Then there is the matter of trying to wean a baby or toddler who is not ready and asks for milk often. When your biological drive tells you to meet your baby's demands there is a strong emotional pull when your baby requests to breastfeed. Prepare to possibly be at odds with your baby on when weaning should happen. Your lactation consultant and peers will often have good suggestions for distraction and encouragement of weaning.

During and after weaning you may experience a form of hormonal depression. Weaning depression is a very real thing, just like postpartum depression. Be prepared to feel big feelings and be sad about drying up, even if it is logical and will over-all make you happier. You may consider weaning more slowly if it impacts you too strongly. If you are prone to depression this is a time to lean on your healthcare team and keep them involved in your current process and changes. You may find you need more support than usual.

Again, be prepared for any hormonal changes when you are weaning—as it is hormonally regulated. You may experience mood shifts, acne, hot flashes, dramatic hair loss, thyroid dysfunction, irregular periods, insomnia, or any other variety of inconveniences.

The physical changes with weaning usually involve feeling engorged off and on as your mammae fill but are not drained. Sometimes they are trying to rebound in supply, to encourage you not to wean. Aches and pains in the breast might persist for months. Your period might return, and it might be irregular for a few months. The breast tissue will involute, and the breast might look flatter and deflated. The breast will internally reconstruct and tighten back up a bit, but this might take years. You are likely to be able to still express small amounts of thick, sticky, salty liquid that is yellow to white for many years, as well.

Bonding and soothing your infant or toddler will change also. Your strategies will change from nursing to other things.

Just like other caregivers, you will continue to bond and nurture them with cuddling, rocking, singing, reading, feeding, and many other methods.

Avoiding Problems, Optimizing Success!

Now, truthfully most parents will only experience a few of these problems, if any. For the majority of parents nursing or pumping does work out fine, especially after the first 4-6 weeks of initiation while you and your baby get to know each other. Much of the initiation is psychological; it is about adjusting to the seemingly constant demands of the newborn. What I want you to take away from this book is not that you need to know everything, but that you do not have to do it alone. There is so much to know about breastfeeding that many have built careers based on breastfeeding medicine!

Most parents experience a few of these problems, and not usually all at once. A particularly challenging breastfeeding relationship experience might entail facing more of these challenges, and a few at the same time. Rarely, a person might face many of these problems simultaneously. Many, if not most, can be worked around, worked through, and overcome. A positive experience is possible, and I think more likely if you go into the process prepared. The first 6 weeks is usually the hardest for most breastfeeding dyads and comes with a steep learning curve. This is when it is essential to have professional and peer support.

Steps you can take to maximize supply

Before Pregnancy get a breast tissue assessment and encourage tissue development. Every time you have a period you have an opportunity during cycles to grow glandular breast tissue. Natural remedies can help encourage this like the herb goat's rue, or wild yam extract which boosts progesterone. Work with someone who knows your medical history and knows natural medicine before you start something like this because even herbs and natural plant extracts are medicine and can be harmful if not used properly.

During Pregnancy you might prepare in the last trimester by taking a prenatal lactation class, doing antenatal hand expression, using natural progesterone creams on the breast (if cleared by your provider), taking goat's rue (if you are deemed low risk and have had your medical clearance to do so), testing for optimal hormone balance, buying a pump, mastering how to use a pump, setting up a nursing station, building a village, and getting a prenatal assessment from an IBCLC. Many people will tell you there is nothing to do while pregnant, but it simply is not true.

Critical to breastfeeding success is plans you make for postpartum while you are pregnant. This means organizing a supportive village. Your modern village will be made up of professionals, friends, and family. Making plans for the early weeks postpartum will give you more emotional and physical energy to devote to healing and breastfeeding. This means making logistical plans around meals and chores. Get creative with ways to minimize your workload and maximize your support. Many families find preparing frozen meals or setting up meal trains to be extremely helpful.

During labor and delivery make sure you have a support team that knows your breastfeeding goals, limit intervention except what is medically necessary, allow intervention when it is lifesaving, have a birth plan that includes your breastfeeding plans and goals. Have a support person present to voice your goals and plans if things start to get de-railed or the team gets distracted.

Immediately postpartum make sure you get a golden hour (barring extreme medical complications), continue with a lot of skin to skin, engage in early removal of milk within an hour after delivery. It is more beneficial to use hand expression when it is colostrum and then switch to pumping once the milk is in.

When your baby is placed skin to skin immediately after delivery one of the main reasons this is helpful, among others, is due to you being able to smell them. Our bodies respond very strongly to stimulation through our olfactory nerves, or our sense of smell. The baby's head is covered in vernix that has a smell that tells your brain that the baby has been born. It reaches the deep primal part of the brain that cannot always be reached or controlled by logic or data. The smells that are emitted from your baby's head continue to play a vital role in bonding and milk making. The reason their scent is so intoxicating is because it is so beneficial to their survival for you to smell them. It releases feel-good hormones, and encourages you to come back for more, and thus be very attentive to and connected with your baby. This can be beneficial for many months for many reasons but is especially critical in the early weeks of establishing milk supply. If you are unable to smell your baby frequently, especially while feeding, then you need to re-create the experience. This can mean smelling their hats and blankets to get the benefits of the scent. You will want to do this as often as possible, but especially while pumping.

During the golden hour you will probably be distracted, or people will attempt to interrupt this process to handle up on other things. Often, while a female is skin to skin with their baby, they will also be delivering placenta and then likely getting stitches; at an incision site for a cesarean or where the vulva was torn if delivered vaginally. Shortly after this is handled one might be encouraged to urinate if you delivered vaginally, to make sure your urethra is intact. Parents who have had a cesarean might have their skin to skin interrupted due to the need to transfer from the operating room back to the recovery room. During the golden hour you will be pressured to do other things or focus on other things. Some people might need to make sure you and baby are stable, and outside of that most things can wait. If the people around you are not respecting your golden hour you can remind them that you want that time protected, or have your partner or doula remind them. You can always ask for tasks to be done later, as long as you and baby are stable. Some things they do for baby might be checking their weight, length, heart rate, respiratory rate, and temperature. They should be able to check some of those things with the baby still on your chest, so do not be afraid to request it if they insist it be done right away.

Immediately postpartum, the first hours of parenting, are often a blur. After laboring and no sleep, and sometimes emergency surgery, you and your partner might be in a half-asleep haze. This is why it is important to learn as much as you can before the baby comes, because what they try to throw at you in your most sleep deprived state will often not stick.

If there are any indicators in the first 2-3 days that baby is not removing milk well, hand expression and pumping will be critical to supply development. If you need to express milk you will need to combine pumping and hand expression, as colostrum is very thick and sticky and not pumped out easily. Clues your baby is not efficiently nursing might be dramatic weight loss, dehydration, low diaper count, hypoglycemia, and jaundice. Some people will encourage you to wait on interventions like this, but until you know your baby nurses efficiently, they can be helpful for long term supply health. If you are unsure that your baby is nursing well or getting enough colostrum, ask for help. If your intuition has you worried despite being encouraged, start hand expressing and supplementing your own milk anyway. You can also start offering donor milk or formula without anyone else's permission. This is your baby; these are your choices.

Usually, in the second or third night babies tend to cry a lot and nurse frequently and for long stretches of time. Many parents are home from the hospital, and without help. It is the most common time for parents to start questioning if baby is getting enough milk. The baby is usually trying very hard to get as much colostrum as possible, and it is also working to get your body to shift into the milk making phase from the colostrum making phase. Unless your baby does not have enough wet diapers, do not let this behavior scare you into supplementing. If you really are doubting things, hand express and spoon feed any milk you can get out as often as you can, and then follow up with an IBCLC within 24 hours.

The early weeks postpartum are when you should be working with an IBCLC, anyway. Frequent milk removal via nursing in the early weeks is most essential to building supply. If your baby does not nurse efficiently it is critical that you pump frequently to drain the breast. Inefficient milk removal might be from a weak or uncoordinated suck, or anatomical anomaly. The brain must get the signal that an infant is surviving and thriving and worthy of making milk for. When it has been a couple weeks if you are still suffering with a low supply then you can explore herbs and medications.

Herbs should be prescribed by an herbalist who knows your medical history. You can easily waste a small fortune on herbs and supplements that claim to boost lactation. It is easy to fall prey to manipulative marketing when you are feeling most vulnerable and working on your supply.

Medications that boost prolactin can also help boost supply but are more controversial. The two available are domperidone and metoclopramide (also called Reglan). As of the writing of this book the FDA in the USA has said domperidone is not safe to use for lactation, but safe for gastrointestinal disease. It is a drug that is used world-wide and in some places over the counter. Depending on where you reside, this might be an option for you, but like with all medications it is not risk free. The most common complaint with domperidone is weight gain. It also has to be weaned off of very slowly to avoid permanent damage to milk making and mood stabilizing receptors. There is also the riskier drug that is more likely to be prescribed in the USA called Reglan (metoclopramide), but many will not prescribe it due it its negative effects on a postpartum parent's mood. Do not be lured by this drug. If you have a low supply, you are high risk for mood disorders and Reglan on top of that exacerbates that risk dramatically.

A good alternative to both is barely water. This is generally widely available and easy to make. Some studies show that it boosts prolactin in the same way as these drugs, without the risky side effects. To me, this is more proof that food is medicine.

For your sanity, try not to fall down the boosting supply rabbit hole. With everything that is available on the internet you will possibly take up dozens of hours of your time just reading through and guessing what to do. This is precious time you could be spending snuggling your baby. Let a professional (or team) help you navigate all of the information and choices. Seek a lactation consultant to help you build a team to support the breastfeeding relationship. Seek an herbalist if you decide to take herbs. Seek body work for you or baby if either of you are tense. You get the idea.

I say often that your baby needs a happy, calm, and connecting parent more than they need breastmilk. Do not sacrifice your sanity or martyr yourself to trying to exclusively breastfeed.

Resources

You should have a healthcare team set up to help you face potential challenges. Start with meeting with an IBCLC. Choose a breastfeeding supportive pediatrician. Ask them questions about what ways they support breastfeeding, and make sure their ideals match yours. Bring in a speech and language pathologist, and myofunctional therapist and body workers like massage therapists, chiropractors and cranial sacral therapists as needed for feeding difficulties. Have an idea of who you would talk to or go see if you feel you needed emotional or mental health support. Ask around your local community for recommendations of these specialists. Build your healthcare village.

Remember that everyone you know is a resource. Your support circle needs to grow, and you should be the one to grow it. Do not wait for people to volunteer, tell them how they can help. When people do offer to help, tell them something specific you want. If someone is willing to do something for you, let them.

Do not forget the amazing resource of technology that we have as modern parents. You can get many free apps on your phone to track feedings, diapers, sleep, measurements, and milestones. You can utilize social media and search engines for many things, as long as you also consult your professional team. Social media can also be very beneficial to combatting isolation and loneliness, as it can connect you with other parents. You can send pictures and video-chat with family if you do not want to have them over, or if they live too far to visit. You can also attend online classes, do online prenatal consults, attend online support groups, and watch how-to videos of many of the hands-on skills you will need like pumping, swaddling, and burping.

You are also a powerful resource unto yourself. You can do a lot to prepare. Go to a prenatal consult. Take the parenting and breastfeeding classes, read the books, do the meal-prep, freeze some padsicles, do the mental and emotional work. Manage your own expectations. Take responsibility for yourself by asking for help and setting boundaries. Give yourself grace, compassion, and patience. Trust your instincts. Seek help early and often.

Find an IBCLC

You need support from a local or virtual IBCLC. When you see a lactation consultant, like myself, I suggest a prenatal lactation assessment to review your risk factors and take steps specific to your risks to maximize your supply before pregnancy, during, and immediately postpartum. They can help in the early weeks and up until weaning, even if that is well into childhood. I, personally, am available for virtual consults and local in-person consults.

Even without some of these problems breastfeeding is generally challenging. Becoming a new parent is challenging. Lean into your community and reach out for help. Do not wait until there is a problem; see an IBCLC before pregnancy, during, and after. Let them monitor your progress in those fragile early weeks. Let them help you troubleshoot, perfect, and optimize your breastfeeding experience.

I am available virtually, find me on Instagram @thelactationpractitioner and I will have the best way to book with me in my bio. Local appointments may be available and might be covered by insurance if you are on the Olympic Peninsula in Washington State.

Utilize your lactation benefits through insurance

The Affordable Healthcare Act, signed into law in 2010, ensures that more females in the United States have access to coverage for lactation support and pumping equipment. As of the writing of this book in 2020, this is still in effect. Health insurance plans, outside of grandfathered plans and certain state Medicaid plans, must provide breastfeeding support and equipment for the duration of breastfeeding, and some help is available during pregnancy. This means you are able to get a prenatal lactation consult, and possibly get your pump before baby comes. The pump provided might be a rental, manual, or electric. Some require birth of the baby before they will issue the pump. It should be up to you and your provider which option is best for you, and they can write a prescription to be filled by a medical supply company. Some plans cover other equipment like bags or valve replacements, or they are at least FSA/HSA (Flexible Spending or Healthcare Spending accounts) eligible. Much of the breastfeeding and pumping paraphernalia is covered under FSA/HSA spending, so always check before you purchase or check if you are eligible for reimbursement. The equipment offered may require partial cost-sharing if you choose to upgrade, but a no-cost option should also be available. The lactation support might need to be with an in-network provider, require prior-authorization, or referral. Lactation services are considered preventative medicine, as lactation is a biological expectation, and you should not have any co-pays, payments toward deductible, or co-insurance fees. If you see an OB/GYN,

CNM, pediatrician, or FNP (like me) who is also an IBCLC you might be covered under preventative medicine as well, and this may not count towards using the lactation consult benefit. This is important to know if your plan places a limit on number of visits per year. This is information you want to clarify while you are still pregnant so you can plan ahead and have help lined up for when you inevitably need it.

Here is a helpful toolkit to help you understand your rights under this law, and suggestions to hold your plan accountable if they are not meeting the standards set forth by the law.

https://www.nwlc.org/sites/default/files/pdfs/
final_nwlcbreastfeedingtoolkit2014_edit.pdf

Find an oral tether/tongue tie provider

If you suspect your child has oral tethers it is best to find a "preferred provider" with a reputation for doing thorough work. Follow up with finding stretches and exercises for oral tethers; you can start these even before a revision. This is where you will want to involve your healthcare village.

https://www.tt-lt-support-network.com/

There are also many Facebook support groups, usually separated by state, where you can get feedback from other parents who have seen providers in your area. They also typically share how their recovery process was, and other associated therapists, consultants, and bodyworkers in the area that aided in their post-procedure recovery and functional optimization.

Infant Risk

This is the resource I mentioned previously for what medication is safe during pregnancy and breastfeeding. They have a website, app, book, and hotline.
https://www.infantrisk.com/

Jack Newman, M.D.
Breastfeeding Medicine Specialist

Jack Newman's website is an excellent resource for breast-feeding information. Visit https://www.breastfeedinginc.ca/

Mother-Baby Behavioral Sleep Lab, University of Notre Dame, Dr. James McKenna

"Safe Infant Sleep" by James J McKenna, Ph.D. https://cosleeping.nd.edu/

PPD/PPA Resources

Postpartum Support International: https://www.postpartum.net/
Warm Line (non-emergent phone support): 1 800 944 4773
Postpartum Support International offers phone support, online chat support, online support meetings and local resources. Online support meetings are held weekly for both moms and dads. Information is available at this site in both English and Spanish.

Text HOME to 741741 if you need immediate assistance you can find help 24 hours a day, 7 days a week and have a cell phone and are in the United States. Their website explains their services. https://www.crisistextline.org/text-us/

Call the National Suicide Prevention Hotline: 1800 273 8255, also available 24/7

Domestic Abuse Resources

National Domestic Violence Hotline, which has a website with education and resources, as well as a chat feature, in addition to their hotline phone number.
https://www.thehotline.org/

When you go to the website you will be prompted with this warning: "Internet usage can be monitored and is impossible to erase completely. If you are concerned your internet usage might be monitored, call us at 1 800 799 SAFE (7233). Learn more about digital security and remember to clear your browser history after visiting this website.
Click the "X" or "Escape" button at any time to leave TheHotline.org immediately."

National Women's Law Center

"Breastfeeding Students" pamphlet FAQs
https://nwlc.org/wp-content/uploads/2016/08/
FAQBreastfeeding_nwlc_PPToolkitAug2016.pdf

Substance Abuse and Mental Health Services Administration

1-800-662-4357
https://www.samhsa.gov/find-help/national-helpline

Final Thoughts

The truth is no matter how much you want to give your child the best and protect them at all costs—you cannot always do that. This is true beyond what happens with breastfeeding. Parenting is filled with times that you must accept that things will not be the way you envisioned. It is one of the harshest realities of parenting. However, I believe we are more plagued if we do not try. If we do not follow our innate instincts to attempt to feed our babies from our bosoms, we do not follow our instincts to protect and nourish physically and emotionally, that is when we put ourselves most at risk.

Being a good parent starts with caring how well you parent. I believe one of our many jobs as parents is to advocate for our children. We do that in part by educating ourselves as much as possible on what an optimal situation might look like and what potential complications might look like. We take the information we learn and push for what we have concluded is best, given our circumstances. This looks quite different for each family, and for each individual child. The options and opinions are many, so you will have to figure out what works for you.

With our first basic task of feeding we can read books and take prenatal classes and meet with IBCLCs. However, I will invite you to remember that you are so much more than a milk maker. A parent provides nourishment in many forms. Parents provide so much more than food to help their babies thrive. You will provide for your baby's basic needs which will teach your baby about love and trust.

It will not matter much when they are adults if they got formula, but it will influence their whole life and personality if you spend their early formative months stressed. If you want to breastfeed: feed the baby, protect your supply, and keep the breast a happy place. Do those three things and then seek help! Seek help early, and often. It is critical to get an evaluation and plan from a professional who knows you and your baby's medical history.

Truthfully, with everything the modern lactating parent faces it seems like we are set up to fail. That is why the USA national rates of initiating are around 79-95% depending on region, but the continuation drops to 20-50% by 6 months. Many cultural messages around breastfeeding make it hard to trust our body. Our culture and our laws do not protect the sacred relationship that is breastfeeding. I hope our culture continues to shift back towards supporting the biological norms of breastfeeding, and the parent-infant dyad's relationship. I hope we continue to see not only the rates of initiation of breastfeeding rise, but the continuation of the breastfeeding relationship at higher rates and for longer stretches of time. I hope that arming more parents with this knowledge I have imparted through this book will contribute to this change.

I implore you not to go into a breastfeeding relationship with hard rules or expectations. Being flexible is what will make you resilient. It will also help preserve your sanity. Be ready for steep and staggering personal growth. When you are pushed to your limits, you will learn your limits. Leave space in your breastfeeding relationship and leave space in your parenting to grieve that which will not come to pass, no matter how much you will it. Managing your expectations for what is realistic and possible will in turn help manage your mental health. Hope for the best and prepare for the worst. Leave space to celebrate what is working and what is enjoyable about the experience. There is always room for the joy and gratitude of what is, and it is also okay to be sad and grieve for what is not. Make room for it all.

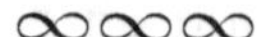

If you enjoyed this book and learned from it, please leave me a
review through the platform that you purchased the book from
and recommend it to your friends. I am also always open to
polite debate and constructive criticism, as I am always seeking
to learn.